RANDOM HOUSE
WEBSTER'S

HANDY

DIET AND
NUTRITION GUIDE

2ND EDITION

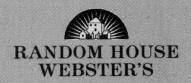

RANDOM HOUSE WEBSTER'S

HANDY

DIET AND NUTRITION GUIDE

2ND EDITION

RANDOM HOUSE
REFERENCE

NEW YORK   TORONTO   LONDON   SYDNEY   AUCKLAND

Acknowledgment

We would like to thank all who helped produce this edition. The expert advice and contributions of Jamie Restler, R.D., C.N.S.D., Clinical Dietitian, Greenwich Hospital, Greenwich, Connecticut, were invaluable. As adviser to the book, Ms. Restler readily shared her expertise in nutrition, particularly in planning the Basic Healthy Diet, Basic Weight Loss, and Special Diets Sections.

Special thanks to Stephen Elliott and Sachem Publishing for editorial services.

Contents

A Word About Nutrition, Health, and Diet

The importance of proper nutrition is universally recognized. It is well established that nutritional factors play a role in at least five of the ten leading causes of death in the United States, including coronary heart disease, stroke, diabetes, certain forms of cancer, and atherosclerosis. The debate over exactly what constitutes a "healthy" diet continues as further discoveries are made almost daily about various nutritional components and well-being. Unfortunately, in recent years, the public has received too many conflicting reports regarding food, nutrition, and health, which has led to confusion and skepticism. Overall, however, the quest for health and wellness has prompted many people to improve their eating habits, exercise regularly, and control their weight.

The purpose of *RHW's Handy Diet and Nutrition Guide,* second edition, is to offer some general guidelines for formulating a diet that is nutritionally sound for most healthy people and to suggest ways to meet special needs associated with certain health problems. The fundamentals of a healthy diet are described and a 7-day meal plan for sensible eating is provided. This same meal plan is also adjusted for a basic weight-loss program of 1,800 or 1,200 calories per day. In addition, there are outlines for diets that alter the amount of sodium, fats, carbohydrate, fiber, lactose, purines, and calcium consumed. Suggestions are made for ensuring the nutritional adequacy of a vegetarian diet. The information provided in this book is built upon the most current and strongest scientific findings available.

This second edition of *RHW's Handy Diet and Nutrition Guide* supplements the diets with information on the Dietary Reference Intakes (DRIs) for vitamins and minerals as well as good food sources for particular nutrients, height and weight standards, calculation of calorie and fat requirements, estimates of calories burned with exercise, how to read a food label, and healthy cooking techniques. The Composition of Foods table covers more than 1,000 separate foods, listing the key nutritional data for a serving of each: calories, protein, fat (total and saturated), cholesterol, carbohydrate (total and fiber), and sodium. This information allows consumers to evaluate the foods being eaten and to develop meal plans based on the guidelines offered in each specific diet.

Nutritional needs are like fingerprints; no two are alike. It is impossible to develop a diet that is perfectly balanced for every individual because nutritional needs are influenced by a variety of factors, including age, sex, body size, activity level, metabolism, medication usage, medical history and health status, and genetic predisposition to various diseases. Therefore, discuss your unique nutritional requirements with a health care provider before beginning any type of diet or regimen. A registered dietitian (R.D.) can help develop an eating plan for good health and wellness.

BASIC HEALTHY DIET

Dietary Guidelines for Americans

The Dietary Guidelines for Americans were revised in 2005 by the U.S. Department of Agriculture and the U.S. Department of Health and Human Services. They reflect the understanding that many common illnesses in American society are related to a diet that is excessive in calories, fat, saturated fat, cholesterol, sodium, and sugar and that lacks complex carbohydrate and fiber. In addition, recommendations are made to define "moderation" in the consumption of alcoholic beverages. While diseases of nutritional deficiency are quite uncommon (in fact many Americans are "overnourished"), some people may not be obtaining an optimal amount of iron and calcium from their diet. The following will help you remain healthy:

ADEQUATE NUTRIENTS

- Consume a variety of nutrient-dense foods and beverages within and among the basic food groups while choosing foods that limit the intake of saturated and *trans* fats, cholesterol, added sugars, salt, and alcohol.

- Meet recommended intakes within energy needs by adopting a balanced eating pattern, such as the U.S. Department of Agriculture (USDA) Food Guide or the Dietary Approaches to Stop Hypertension (DASH) Eating Plan.

WEIGHT MANAGEMENT

- To maintain body weight in a healthy range, balance calories from foods and beverages with calories expended.

- To prevent gradual weight gain over time, make small decreases in food and beverage calories and increase physical activity.

PHYSICAL ACTIVITY

- Engage in regular physical activity and reduce sedentary activities to promote health, psychological well-being, and a healthy body weight.

  - To reduce the risk of chronic disease in adulthood: Engage in at least 30 minutes of moderate-intensity physical activity, above usual activity, at work or home on most days of the week.

- For most people, greater health benefits can be obtained by engaging in physical activity of more vigorous intensity or longer duration.

- To help manage body weight and prevent gradual, unhealthy body weight gain in adulthood: Engage in approximately 60 minutes of moderate- to vigorous-intensity activity on most days of the week while not exceeding caloric intake requirements.

- To sustain weight loss in adulthood: Participate in at least 60 to 90 minutes of daily moderate-intensity physical activity while not exceeding caloric intake requirements. Some people may need to consult with a healthcare provider before participating in this level of activity.

- Achieve physical fitness by including cardiovascular conditioning, stretching exercises for flexibility, and resistance exercises or calisthenics for muscle strength and endurance.

HEALTHY FOODS
- Consume a sufficient amount of fruits and vegetables while staying within energy needs. Two cups of fruit and 2½ cups of vegetables per day are recommended for a reference 2,000-calorie intake, with higher or lower amounts depending on the calorie level.

- Choose a variety of fruits and vegetables each day. In particular, select from all five vegetable subgroups (dark green, orange, legumes, starchy vegetables, and other vegetables) several times a week.

- Consume 3 or more ounce-equivalents of whole-grain products per day, with the rest of the recommended grains coming from enriched or whole-grain products. In general, at least half the grains should come from whole grains.

- Consume 3 cups per day of fat-free or low-fat milk or equivalent milk products.

FATS
- Consume less than 10% of calories from saturated fatty acids and less than 300 mg/day of cholesterol, and keep *trans* fatty acid consumption as low as possible.

- Keep total fat intake between 20%–35% percent of calories, with most fats coming from sources of polyunsaturated and monounsaturated fatty acids, such as fish, nuts, and vegetable oils.

- When selecting and preparing meat, poultry, dry beans, and milk or milk products, make choices that are lean, low-fat, or fat-free.

- Limit intake of fats and oils high in saturated and/or *trans* fatty acids, and choose products low in such fats and oils.

CARBOHYDRATES

- Choose fiber-rich fruits, vegetables, and whole grains often.

- Choose and prepare foods and beverages with little added sugars or caloric sweeteners, such as amounts suggested by the USDA Food Guide and the DASH Eating Plan.

- Reduce the incidence of dental caries by practicing good oral hygiene and consuming sugar- and starch-containing foods and beverages less frequently.

SODIUM AND POTASSIUM

- Consume less than 2,300 mg (approximately 1 teaspoon of salt) of sodium per day.

- Choose and prepare foods with little salt. At the same time, consume potassium-rich foods, such as fruits and vegetables.

ALCOHOLIC BEVERAGES

- Those who choose to drink alcoholic beverages should do so sensibly and in moderation—defined as the consumption of up to one drink per day for women and up to two drinks per day for men.

- Alcoholic beverages should not be consumed by some individuals, including those who cannot restrict their alcohol intake, women of childbearing age who may become pregnant, pregnant and lactating women, children and adolescents, individuals taking medications that can interact with alcohol, and those with specific medical conditions.

- Alcoholic beverages should be avoided by individuals engaging in activities that require attention, skill, or coordination, such as driving or operating machinery.

6

FOOD SAFETY
- To avoid microbial food-borne illness:
  - Clean hands, food contact surfaces, and fruits and vegetables. Meat and poultry should not be washed or rinsed.
  - Separate raw, cooked, and ready-to-eat foods while shopping, preparing, or storing foods.
  - Cook foods to a safe temperature to kill microorganisms.
  - Chill (refrigerate) perishable food promptly and defrost foods properly.
  - Avoid raw (unpasteurized) milk or any products made from unpasteurized milk, raw or partially cooked eggs or foods containing raw eggs, raw or undercooked meat and poultry, unpasteurized juices, and raw sprouts.

MyPyramid

The USDA has developed new guidelines to help Americans choose a healthy diet and active lifestyle. MyPyramid (which replaced the original Food Guide Pyramid) encourages balancing caloric intake with daily physical activity, and consuming a diet rich in a variety of nutrient-dense foods while limiting saturated and *trans* fats, cholesterol, added sugars, salt, and alcohol. The recommended number of daily servings from each food group depends on age, gender, and activity level. A personal profile can be developed at: www.mypyramid.gov.

Grains: In order to maintain a diet low in fat, high in complex carbohydrate and fiber, and full of vitamins and minerals (several B vitamins, iron, magnesium, and selenium), the highest number of servings per day should be from this group. These foods are not fattening if the right selections are made and portion sizes are monitored. Use only a small amount of fat and sugar when preparing grains or as spreads and limit most baked goods, such as cakes, cookies, doughnuts, pastries, and pies. About 50% of choices from this group should be whole grain to ensure adequate fiber intake. Daily recommendation: approximately 5–8 oz equivalents (3–4 oz equivalents from whole grains).

1 oz equivalent: 1 slice bread; 1 "mini" bagel; ½ hamburger roll or English muffin; 1 cup cold cereal; ½ cup cooked hot cereal, rice, or pasta; 1 tortilla (6″ diameter); or 1 pancake (4½″ diameter).

Vegetables: Vegetables are excellent sources of fiber; vitamins A, C, and E; potassium; and folate, and generally low in calories and fat. Serve and prepare vegetables with a minimal amount of butter, margarine, oil, sauce, or salad dressing (count these additions as fat). Daily recommendation: approximately 2–3 cups per day (weekly totals: approximately 2–3 cups dark green, 1½–2 cups orange, 2½–3 cups dried beans and peas, and 5½–7 cups other vegetables).

1 cup serving: 2 cups raw green leafy vegetables; 1 cup cooked or raw other vegetables; 1 cup vegetable juice; 1 medium baked potato; 1 cup dry beans or peas.*

Fruits: Fruits are also excellent sources of fiber, vitamin C, potassium, and folate, and low in calories, fat, and sodium. Whole fruits usually have more fiber than fruit juice. To keep sugar content low, drink 100% fruit juice instead of punch, fruit-flavored drinks, or soda (which count as sweets) and purchase canned fruits in their own juice. Daily recommendation: approximately 1½–2 cups.

1 cup serving: 1 cup fruit or 100% fruit juice; ½ cup dried fruit; 1 large banana, orange, or peach; 1 medium pear or grapefruit; 1 small apple.

Milk: Milk, yogurt, and cheese provide calcium, potassium, vitamin D, and protein. Because these foods can supply saturated fat and cholesterol, choose 1% fat or nonfat milk and yogurt and low-fat or "part skim" cheeses. Cottage cheese is lower in calcium than other cheeses. Ice cream contains more sugar but less calcium than most of the other choices in this group. For lactose intolerance, choose lactose-reduced or low lactose options or try taking lactase enzyme before consuming milk products. Daily recommendation: 3 cups.

1 cup serving: 1 cup milk or yogurt; 2 oz. processed cheese; 1½ oz. natural cheese; ½ cup ricotta cheese; 2 cups cottage cheese; 1 cup frozen yogurt; 1½ cups ice cream.

*If daily protein needs are met with animal sources, count beans and peas as a vegetable. If intake of animal protein is limited, count beans and peas as a meat.

8

Meat and Beans: Meat, poultry, fish, eggs, dry beans and peas, nuts, and seeds supply protein, iron, zinc, magnesium, B vitamins (thiamin, riboflavin, niacin, B6), and vitamin E. Animal foods tend to be high in saturated fat and cholesterol. Therefore, choose more fish, nuts, and seeds to help ensure most of the daily fat allowance (20–35% of calories) is unsaturated. Limit saturated fat by choosing skinless poultry and lean cuts of red meat such as flank, round, or sirloin steak, extra-lean ground beef, center loin or tenderloin pork, and leg of lamb or loin chops. Trim all visible fat and avoid frying. Eat organ meats infrequently and limit egg yolks to 3–4 per week. Use dry beans and peas as an entrée for maximum fiber and no saturated fat or cholesterol. Daily recommendation: approximately 5–6½ oz. equivalents.

1 oz equivalent: 1 oz. cooked lean meat, poultry, fish, or shellfish; 1 egg; 1 Tbsp. peanut butter; ½ oz. nuts or seeds; ¼ cup cooked dry beans or peas.*

Oils: This group includes fats from plants and fish that are liquid at room temperature. Oils provide essential fatty acids and vitamin E. Oils also supply calories and should be used in moderation. Choices include canola, corn, cottonseed, olive, safflower, soybean, and sunflower oil; soft margarine (*trans fat*-free); mayonnaise; and salad dressings. Daily allowance: approximately 5–7 tsp.

Discretionary calories: Once "essential" calories have been met by choosing low-fat, low-sugar items from each food group, there may be room for treats within a calorie limit. Discretionary calories include solid fats (butter, cheese, whole milk, ice cream, well-marbled cuts of meats), added sugars (soda, candy, cakes, cookies, pies), and alcohol. Generally, allowances are only 100–300 calories daily.

Physical activity: This is a key component of MyPyramid and promotes weight management, strength and endurance, reduced risk of chronic disease, and a sense of well-being. Moderate to vigorous activity is recommended most days of the week for at least 30 minutes for health, 60 minutes to prevent weight gain, and 60–90 minutes for weight loss. At least 10 minutes of physical activity at a time is sufficient and can accumulate throughout the day. Include aerobic activity (brisk walking, jog-

*If daily protein needs are met with animal sources, count beans and peas as a vegetable. If intake of animal protein is limited, count beans and peas as a meat.

ging, swimming, cycling), stretching or yoga, and resistance (weight lifting).

Reading Food Labels

The Food and Drug Administration requires by law that nearly all processed foods have a "Nutrition Facts" panel on their packaging. This standard format allows one to identify the exact content of many nutrients and to better understand how to fit that food into an overall diet. Here are some important points about food labeling.

1. The place to start when you look at the Nutrition Facts label is the *Serving Size* and the number of servings in the package. Serving sizes are standardized to make it easier to compare similar foods. They are provided in familiar units, such as cups of pieces, followed by the metric amount—the number of grams.

2. The Nutrient Content is provided for Calories, Protein, Total Fat, Saturated Fat, Cholesterol, Carbohydrates, Fiber, and Sodium. These nutrients were chosen because of their strong link to many diseases afflicting Americans.

3. The Percentage (%) Daily Value indicates what portion of the recommended Daily Value (DV) is met by one serving of that food item for a person who needs 2,000 calories a day. Based upon calorie needs, one can determine the DV numbers for Total Fat (30% calories), Saturated Fat (10% calories), Carbohydrates (60% calories), and Protein (10% calories). Use the resources in the book as a start or seek the assistance of a registered dietitian. For other nutrients, the DVs are the same for everyone, including cholesterol (goal: 300 mg or less daily), sodium (goal: no more than 2,400 mg), and fiber (goal: at least 25 grams a day). In addition, the % DV is provided for vitamins A and C as well as for calcium and iron. A 5% DV or less is considered low, whereas 20% DV or more is considered high for all nutrients.

4. *Trans Fat* is created through the hydrogenation of liquid oils to form a solid (as in shortening and hard margarines). It is found in processed foods, including crackers, candies, cookies, snack foods, fried foods, and baked goods. Consumption of trans fat increases the risk of coronary heart disease. It is therefore recommended to keep intake of trans fats as

low as possible. Food companies and restaurants are making efforts to reduce or remove trans fat from products and recipes.

5. If a food product meets certain strict criteria, a nutrient claim may appear on the label. The claim gives a general idea of the amount of the nutrient in the product per serving, but it is always best to look at the Nutrition Facts panel for more details. The following terms are allowed:

Free	There is virtually none of the nutrient stated per serving. Per serving: less than 5 calories; less than 0.5 g total fat, saturated fat, and trans fat; less than 2 mg cholesterol; less than 5 mg sodium; less than 0.5 g sugars.
Low	The meaning varies for each nutrient. Per serving there can be no more than 140 mg sodium (low-sodium); 3 gm total fat (low-fat); 1 gm saturated fat (low saturated fat); 20 mg cholesterol (low-cholesterol); 40 calories (low-calorie).
Very Low	Applies to sodium only. Means no more than 35 mg sodium per serving.
Reduced or less	Contains 25% less of the nutrient stated (fat, sodium, or calories) than the regular version or comparable product.
Light or lite	Contains 50% less fat or sodium or ⅓ less calories than the regular version or comparable product.
% Fat Free	When "low-fat" requirement is met. The percentage of fat present by weight (not by percentage of calories from fat).
Lean	Meat or poultry products containing less than 10 gm fat, 4 gm saturated fat, and 95 mg cholesterol per 3.5 ounce portion (deck of cards size).
Extra-Lean	Meat, poultry, or seafood products containing less than 5 gm fat, 2 gm saturated fat, and 95 mg cholesterol per serving).
Good Source	Provides 10–19% Daily Value for the nutrient stated (fiber, calcium, vitamin A or C).
Excellent Source	Provides at least 20% Daily Value for the nutrient stated (fiber, calcium, vitamin A or C).

6. When there is a strong relationship between a nutrient or food component and health, a health claim may appear on the label. The product must meet certain criteria for such claims to be allowed.

Dietary Reference Intakes

Dietary Reference Intakes (DRIs) include the Recommended Dietary Allowances (RDAs) and the Adequate Intakes (AIs) for selected nutrients. These values aim to prevent deficiencies and reduce the risk of chronic diseases. The RDA is the average level of intake that will meet the nutritional needs of most healthy people. For some nutrients, there is not enough scientific information to establish an RDA, so only an estimated adequate intake is listed, a recommended intake level assumed to be adequate.

Vitamins and Minerals

The following lists indicate those foods that are especially high in specific vitamins and minerals. A balanced diet should provide sufficient amounts of these nutrients.

VITAMINS

Vitamin A
Beneficial to vision, reproduction, growth, immune function; mucous membranes, bone, skin, and teeth need vitamin A for proper development and maintenance. Beta-carotene, a precursor of vitamin A found in some fruits and vegetables, functions as an antioxidant.

> Cereals (fortified)
> Eggs
> Fruits (especially apricots, cantaloupe, mangoes, papaya, peaches)
> Organ meats (liver)
> Margarine
> Milk
> Vegetables (broccoli, carrots, collard greens, kale, pumpkin,
>   spinach, sweet potato, sweet red pepper, winter squash)

B-complex
These vitamins are all necessary for the proper metabolism of carbohydrate, protein, and fat. They are also needed for normal functioning of

Dietary Reference Intakes (DRIs)
Recommended Vitamin and Mineral Intakes for Individuals

Life Stage Group	Children 1–3 y	4–8 y	Males 9–13 y	14–18 y	19–50 y
VITAMINS					
Vit A (mcg/d)	300	400	600	900	900
Vit C (mcg/d)	15	25	45	75	90
Vit D (mcg/d)	5	5	5	5	5
Vit E (mg/d)	6	7	11	15	15
Vit K (mcg/d)	30	55	60	75	120
Thiamine (mg/d	0.5	0.6	0.9	1.2	1.2
Riboflavin (mg/d)	0.5	0.6	0.9	1.3	1.3
Niacin (mg/d)	6	8	12	16	16
Vit B-6 (mg/d)	0.5	0.6	1.0	1.3	1.3
Folate (mcg/d)	150	200	300	400	400
Vit B-12 (mcg/d)	0.9	1.2	1.8	2.4	2.4
MINERALS					
Calcium (mg/d)	500	800	1,300	1,300	1,000
Iodine (mcg/d)	90	90	120	150	150
Iron (mg/d)	7	10	8	11	8
Magnesium (mg/d)	80	130	240	410	400
Phosphorus (mg/d)	460	500	1,250	1,250	700
Selenium (mcg/d)	20	30	40	55	55
Zinc (mg/d)	3	5	8	11	11

Estimated Adequate Intakes (AIs) for adults of various vitamins and minerals:

Biotin	30 mcg	Fluoride	3.0–4.0 mg
Chromium	20–35 mcg	Pantothenic Acid	5.0 mg
Copper	900 mcg		

Estimated AIs for healthy adults:

Potassium	4.7 g	Sodium	1.5 g

the nervous, muscular, and cardiovascular, and digestive systems and for maintenance of skin, nails, and hair.

Thiamine (B1)
Beef (lean)
Breads and cereals (whole grain, enriched or fortified)
Dried beans, peas
Eggs
Fish

51–70 y	Over 70 y	Females 9–13	14–18	19–50	51–70	Over 70
900	900	600	700	700	700	700
90	90	45	65	75	75	75
10	15	5	5	5	10	15
15	15	11	15	15	15	15
120	120	60	75	90	90	90
1.2	1.2	0.9	1.0	1.1	1.1	1.1
1.3	1.3	0.9	1.0	1.1	1.1	1.1
16	16	12	14	14	14	14
1.7	1.7	1.0	1.2	1.3	1.5	1.5
400	400	300	400	400	400	400
2.4	2.4	1.8	2.4	2.4	2.4	2.4
1,200	1,200	1,300	1,300	1,000	1,200	1,200
150	150	120	150	150	150	150
8	8	8	15	18	8	8
420	420	240	360	320	320	320
700	700	1,250	1,250	700	700	700
55	55	40	55	55	55	55
11	11	8	9	8	8	8

Note: This table presents Recommended Dietary Allowances (RDAs) in **bold type** and Adequate Intakes (AIs) in regular type. RDAs and AIs may both be used as goals for individual intake. RDAs are set to meet the needs of almost all (97–98%) individuals in a group. AIs are believed to cover the needs of all individuals in the group, but lack of data or uncertainty in the data prevents being able to specify with confidence the percentage of individuals covered by this intake. The full tables for Dietary Reference Intakes (DRIs) may be accessed at: http://www.iom.edu/Object.File/Master/21/372/0.pdf.

    Nuts
    Organ meats
    Pork and ham
    Rice
    Wheat germ

Riboflavin (B2)
    Bread and cereals (enriched or fortified)
    Cheese

Eggs
Fish
Legumes
Liver
Meat
Milk
Nuts
Pork
Yogurt
Vegetables (asparagus, broccoli, and spinach)
Wheat germ

Niacin (B3)

Beans
Beef
Cereals (enriched or fortified)
Dairy
Fish (especially salmon, swordfish, tuna)
Legumes
Liver (organ meats)
Nuts and peanut butter
Poultry

Pyridoxine (B6)

Avocado
Bananas
Beans (especially garbanzo, lima, and soy)
Beef
Cereals (fortified/whole grain)
Eggs
Fish (especially halibut, salmon, tuna)
Nuts (especially peanut butter, filberts, walnuts)
Organ meats (liver)
Pork
Potatoes
Poultry
Prunes
Spinach
Sunflower seeds
Whole grains

Cobalamin (B12)
Found only in animal foods.

- Beef
- Cheese
- Eggs
- Fish (especially haddock, salmon, trout, tuna)
- Fortified breakfast cereals
- Lamb
- Milk
- Organ meats (liver, kidney)
- Pork
- Poultry
- Shellfish (especially clams, crab, lobster, oysters, mussels)
- Yogurt

Pantothenic Acid

- Chicken
- Egg yolk
- Fish (especially salmon, trout, tuna)
- Lean meats
- Legumes
- Liver, kidney
- Milk
- Oatmeal
- Shellfish
- Vegetables (especially broccoli, cauliflower, corn, mushrooms, potatoes, sweet potatoes)
- Whole grains

Folate
Necessary for synthesis of red blood cells and for functioning of the nervous and gastrointestinal systems. Also may promote heart health. Prevents certain birth defects.

- Beans (garbanzo, lima, pinto) and peas
- Cereals (fortified/whole grain)
- Eggs
- Legumes
- Liver
- Nuts
- Oranges, bananas

Vegetables (especially asparagus, broccoli, mustard and turnip greens, romaine lettuce, spinach)

Biotin
Beneficial to circulation and integrity of hair and skin. Needed for metabolism of foods.

Cereals
Egg yolk
Fish
Nuts
Organ meats (liver, kidney)
Soy flour
Wheat bran

Vitamin C
Needed for healing of wounds and maintaining healthy bones and teeth. Enhances iron absorption. Controversial as to whether it helps prevent or speed recovery from the common cold. Functions as an antioxidant.

Cereals (fortified only)
Fruits and fruit juices (especially cantaloupe, grapefruit, honeydew, kiwi, lemon, mango, orange, pineapple, raspberries, strawberries, tangerine)
Potatoes (sweet and white, baked)
Vegetables (especially broccoli, Brussels sprouts, cabbage, cauliflower, collard greens, kale, green or red pepper, mustard greens, rutabaga, spinach, tomatoes and tomato juice, turnip greens)

Note: Cook vegetables in a minimum amount of water or steam them to retain as much vitamin C as possible.

Vitamin D
Necessary for proper bone development and maintenance. Helps with absorption of calcium. Regulates calcium and phosphorus levels in the blood. The body can manufacture Vitamin D from exposure to 10–15 minutes of sunlight per day.

Cod liver oil
Eggs
Fish (especially, herring, mackerel, salmon, sardines, tuna)

Liver
Margarine (fortified)
Milk (fortified)
Oysters
Pudding and custard (prepared with vitamin D milk)
Shellfish (especially oysters, shrimp)

Vitamin E
*Primary function is to act as an antioxidant that protects body tissues from damage. May be protective against cancer, **but studies are not conclusive.***

Fish (especially herring, mackerel, salmon, sardines)
Fortified cereal
Mangos
Mayonnaise
Nuts and peanut butter
Olives
Salad dressing
Shellfish (oysters, shrimp)
Sunflower seeds
Vegetables (green leafy varieties, primarily: asparagus, avocado, broccoli, collard greens, dandelion greens, spinach, sweet potatoes, turnip greens)
Vegetable oils
Wheat germ

Vitamin K
Plays an important role in blood clotting and bone mineralization.

Green leafy vegetables (especially broccoli, Brussels sprouts, cabbage, collard greens, kale, lettuce, [green leaf, romaine, iceberg, endive], mustard greens, parsley [raw], spinach, Swiss chard, turnip greens)
Soybean oil

MINERALS

Calcium
Major function is development and maintenance of bones and teeth. Also beneficial to blood clotting, heart, and nervous system. May play a role in weight management. Primarily derived from dairy products, but some other foods below are notable sources.

Cereal (if fortified with calcium)
Cheese
Fish (those with bone consumed such as canned salmon, sardines)
Ice cream and ice milk
Milk
Orange juice (if fortified with calcium)
Pudding and custard
Tofu (if made with calcium sulfate)
Vegetables, certain (bok choy, broccoli, collard greens, kale, mustard greens, turnip greens)
Yogurt (including frozen yogurt)

Chromium

Essential for the metabolism of foods, especially carbohydrates, and for blood sugar control.

Apples, bananas
Bran
Brewer's yeast
Broccoli
Chicken/turkey
Eggs
Liver
Meats
Potatoes
Whole grain breads and cereals

Copper

Necessary for many metabolic processes. Facilitates the functions of iron. Promotes healthy bones. Possible antioxidant properties.

Cereal (wheat bran)
Legumes
Liver
Mushrooms
Nuts and seeds
Shellfish (especially oysters)
Whole grains

Fluoride

Important for development and maintenance of bones and teeth.

Fish with bones

Foods and beverages prepared with fluoridated water
Tea
Water (if fluoridated)

Iodine
Essential for production of thyroid hormones and energy metabolism.
Fish (saltwater varieties)
Salt (iodized)
Seafood
Seaweed

Iron
Beneficial to red blood cell production and the immune system. Necessary for oxygen transport to cells.
Beans
Cereals (bran, whole grain or fortified)
Dried fruit (apricots, prunes, raisins)
Fish
Legumes (beans and peas)
Liver
Molasses (blackstrap)
Nuts and seeds
Poultry
Sardines
Shellfish (clams, oysters)
Spinach
Tofu

Magnesium
Needed for normal cardiac, neurologic, and immune functioning. Maintains strong bones. Helps regulate blood sugar and blood pressure. Important for energy metabolism and protein synthesis.
Avocado
Banana
Bread (if whole grain)
Cereals (bran and whole grain)
Halibut
Legumes (beans and peas)
Molasses (blackstrap)
Nuts and seeds

Potato
Spinach
Tofu

Phosphorus

Essential for development and maintenance of teeth and bones, muscle and nerve function, and energy metabolism.

Beans, peas
Breads and cereals (whole grain or enriched)
Cheese
Eggs
Fish and shellfish (especially clams, crab, flounder, lobster, scallops, shrimp)
Meats
Milk
Nuts and seeds
Poultry

Potassium

An electrolyte integral to fluid balance and to muscle and nerve function. May help lower high blood pressure.

Beans
Cereals (bran)
Fish and shellfish (especially cod, flounder, salmon)
Fruits (especially apricots, bananas, cantaloupes, dates, grapefruit juice, honeydew, nectarines, oranges, prunes, raisins)
Meats and poultry
Milk and milk products
Nuts and peanut butter
Potatoes (sweet, white)
Vegetables (especially asparagus, avocado, beet greens, broccoli, Brussels sprouts, carrots, cooked chard, collard greens, corn, peas, pumpkin, spinach, sweet potatoes, tomatoes and tomato products, winter squash)

Note: In order to preserve potassium content, steam vegetables and do not boil potatoes.

Selenium

Has antioxidant properties. Supports thyroid function and immune system.

Beef

Fish and shellfish (cod, tuna)
Garlic
Nuts and seeds
Organ meats
Poultry
Wheat germ

Zinc
Beneficial to the metabolism of protein, carbohydrates, and fat. Supports healthy immune system, wound healing, sense of taste and smell, normal growth and development.

Beans, peas
Beef (lean)
Cereals (bran, whole grain or fortified)
Cheese (Swiss)
Lamb
Liver
Milk and milk products
Nuts
Pork
Poultry (especially dark meat)
Shellfish (especially clams, crab, oysters)

Nutritional Supplements

Each year, consumers spend billions of dollars on nutritional supplements. Many people are looking for increased energy and vitality, while others have heard that large doses of a certain vitamin, mineral, or food supplement will prevent or cure a particular disease. The truth is that a person who is healthy and who eats a balanced diet should be getting the amount of vitamins and minerals needed according to the Dietary Reference Intakes (DRIs). Obtaining vitamins and minerals from food is best because other nutrients, such as complex carbohydrates, fiber, and protein, are also obtained. A vitamin or mineral supplement is appropriate under some circumstances:

- When you do not eat the recommended number of servings from one or more food groups in the MyPyramid for an extended period of time whether due to a hectic lifestyle, food preferences, or personal beliefs. Many women do not consume enough servings from the dairy group to get the required amount of calcium. Strict vegetarians are at risk for several deficiencies, including vitamins B12, D, and riboflavin as well as calcium, iron, and zinc.

- Pregnant or lactating women need more iron, folate, and calcium. Prenatal supplements are recommended by many physicians.

- Diets that contain fewer than 1,200 calories a day, even when very well planned, will, most likely, lack one or more nutrients.

If a nutritional supplement is taken, read labels and find one that provides no more than 100% of the Recommended Daily Allowance (RDA) for vitamins and minerals. Doses of vitamins and minerals far beyond the RDA can be dangerous and should not exceed Tolerable Upper Intake Levels (ULs), especially for the fat-soluble vitamins A, D, E, and K. The saying "If some is good, more is better" does not apply to nutrition.

What of claims that high doses of a particular nutrient or nutritional supplement can ward off or treat diseases? Claims are made that vitamin C helps the common cold, that vitamin E prevents heart disease and cancer, and that fish oils, garlic, or niacin lower cholesterol levels. While there have been new and promising research findings about many nutrients and supplements, do not confuse these with a recommendation to start taking all sorts of pills, potions, and powders. Often, the dosages required are so high that, without the supervision of your physician, more harm than good can be done. Always ask your doctor before taking any nutritional supplements.

7-DAY MENU PLAN: Basic Healthy Diet

The following menu plan conforms to the 2005 Dietary Guidelines for Americans and consists of approximately 2,000 calories. Foods generally thought of as "bad" (because they are somewhat high in fat, sodium, or sugar) can be incorporated into a diet if these choices are exercised in moderation and balanced by more nutritious selections. Depending upon food preferences and individual calorie needs, adjust the menus accordingly by using the Composition of Foods table (page 63) as a guide. To reduce the calories in this plan, consider eliminating the desserts and sweets; reducing the amount of added fats or using reduced fat versions of salad dressings, mayonnaise, or margarine; and eating smaller portions of most foods. For those who need to eat more calories, there is room for larger serving sizes, but try to avoid too many sweets and added fats.

Note: All margarine is tub form from corn oil. Oils used in food preparation are preferably canola, olive, or corn. The portion sizes listed for meat, fish, poultry, rice, stuffing, hot cereal, and hot vegetables are based on weight or cup measurement after cooking. Beverages such as plain coffee or tea, water, and sugar-free beverages have negligible nutritional value and can be used freely. The meal plan can be adjusted to include other beverages such as soft drinks or juice.

SUNDAY
Breakfast
- 3 pancakes, grilled using about 1 tsp. canola oil and topped with 1 Tbsp. tub margarine and 3 Tbsp. maple syrup
- 2 strips bacon
- 1 cup fresh fruit salad
- 1 cup 1% fat milk

Lunch
Hamburger:
- 3 ounces extra-lean ground beef, broiled
- 1 Tbsp. catsup
- Lettuce and tomato
- Whole wheat bun
- 10 oven-baked steak fries with 1 Tbsp. catsup
- 1 cup low-fat fruit yogurt

Dinner
- 3 ounces roasted or grilled chicken breast, no skin
- 1 cup steamed asparagus
- 1 cup wild rice
- 1 large orange

Snacks and Treats
- 1 cup 1% fat milk
- 2 graham cracker squares

MONDAY
Breakfast
- ½ grapefruit
- 1 whole wheat bagel

2 Tbsp. peanut butter
1 cup 1% milk

Lunch

Tuna salad sandwich:
 ½ cup canned light tuna with celery and 1 Tbsp. mayonnaise
 Lettuce and tomato
 2 slices pumpernickel bread
1 cup low-fat fruit yogurt
1 large peach

Dinner

3 ounces roast pork, trimmed
½ cup unsweetened applesauce
1 cup steamed broccoli
1 medium baked potato
2 tsp. tub margarine

Snacks and Treats

1 cup 1% fat milk
4 fig bar cookies

TUESDAY
Breakfast

½ grapefruit
1 bran muffin
1 Tbsp. jam
1 cup 1% fat milk

Lunch

Turkey sandwich:
 3 oz. turkey breast
 Lettuce and tomato
 2 tsp. honey mustard
 2 slices whole wheat bread
¾ cup baby carrots
1 large apple

Dinner

2 cups mixed green salad with 2 Tbsp. vinaigrette dressing

Spaghetti with meatballs:

    2 cups cooked spaghetti noodles

    2 medium meatballs (about 3 ounces extra-lean ground beef)

    ¾ cup marinara sauce

    2 Tbsp. low-sodium Parmesan cheese

Snacks and Treats

1 cup low-fat fruit yogurt

½ ounce sunflower seeds, hulled

WEDNESDAY
Breakfast

1 whole wheat English muffin

1 Tbsp. jam

1 scrambled egg, using about 1 tsp. tub margarine and 1% fat milk

1 cup 1% fat milk

Lunch

Chef's salad:

    2 cups mixed greens

    1 medium tomato, quartered

    1 ounce roast beef

    1 ounce turkey

    1 ounce low-sodium Swiss cheese

    2 Tbsp. Italian dressing

4 sesame bread sticks

20 grapes

Dinner

Tofu stir-fry:

    2 tsp. canola oil

    ¾ cup tofu (about 6 ounces)

    1½ cup mixed vegetables such as pea pods, carrots, bean
        sprouts, mushrooms, broccoli, baby corn, water chestnuts

    2 Tbsp. reduced-sodium soy sauce

1 cup brown rice

3 pineapple slices in own juice

Snacks and Treats

1 cup 1% fat milk

4 gingersnap cookies

THURSDAY
Breakfast
>1 cup oatmeal
>1 Tbsp. honey
>1 large banana
>1 cup 1% fat milk

Lunch
>Roast beef sandwich:
>>3 ounces roast beef
>>Lettuce and tomato
>>2 tsp. mustard
>>2 slices rye bread
>
>1 cup coleslaw
>1 cup honeydew melon

Dinner
>Turkey chili:
>>3 ounces ground turkey
>>½ cup kidney or pinto beans
>>½ cup low-sodium diced tomatoes
>>½ cup barley
>>¼ cup shredded low-sodium cheddar cheese
>
>1 small piece of cornbread

Snacks and Treats
>1 cup low-fat fruit yogurt

FRIDAY
Breakfast
>1 cup bran flake cereal
>¾ cup strawberries
>1 cup 1% fat milk

Lunch
>1 bowl lentil soup
>2 slices multigrain bread
>2 ounces low-sodium Swiss cheese
>1 cup tomato and cucumber salad with vinaigrette dressing
>1 medium pear

Dinner
3 ounces baked or broiled trout
1 large baked sweet potato
1½ cup stir-fried green beans with almonds (1 Tbsp. chopped
 blanched almonds, 1 tsp. olive oil)

Snacks and Treats
1 small piece homemade blueberry pie (⅛th of a 9-inch pie), using
 vegetable shortening in crust)
1 cup 1% fat milk

SATURDAY
Breakfast
Mushroom, onion, and pepper egg-white omelet, prepared with 1
 tsp. canola oil and 4 egg whites
2 slices whole wheat toast
2 tsp. tub margarine
1 cup cantaloupe
1 cup 1% fat milk

Lunch
Chicken vegetable stew:
 3 ounces stewed chicken
 1 cup mixed vegetables (carrots, green beans, corn, potatoes,
 onions, celery)
1 cup whole wheat egg noodles
1 cup low-fat fruit yogurt

Dinner
2 cups tossed salad with 2 Tbsp. vinaigrette dressing
2 slices cheese pizza from large pie
1 cup cranberry-apple juice

Snacks and Treats
2 plums

BASIC WEIGHT LOSS

General recommendations for a sensible weight-loss diet resemble the guidelines for a healthy, balanced diet. They involve eating a variety of foods but reducing the overall number of calories consumed. The easiest way to accomplish this is by eating fewer foods that are high in fat and/or sugar content and by limiting alcohol, which can be a substantial source of empty calories. Also, concentrate on eating more fiber, including whole grains, fruits, and vegetables. Most of these foods are naturally low in fat and calorie content. In addition, increasing fiber will add bulk to the diet and will help to provide a feeling of fullness. Choose more skinless poultry, fish, and dried beans and peas because they usually contain less fat (especially saturated fat) and calories than most cuts of beef, pork, or lamb. Dairy products should be low- or nonfat to save on calories and fat.

Solid fats such as butter, cheese, and whole milk should be used very sparingly. Try to bake, broil, grill, poach, or steam foods instead of frying them. To sauté items without extra fat and calories, use a non-stick skillet and vegetable cooking spray. To add flavor and variety to foods, use a splash of lemon or lime juice, garlic, spices, and herbal vinegar instead of calorie- and fat-laden gravies and sauces. For dessert, try fresh fruit, sugar-free gelatin, graham crackers, and low-fat frozen yogurt. But remember that low-fat or fat-free frozen desserts and baked goods can be a substantial source of calories that should be counted into your total calorie allotment. Beverages may also contribute calories to your diet. Drink as many calorie-free liquids as possible.

Budget calories by eating a little less at some meals to allow for extra calories at parties and special occasions. However, do not skip meals. Be sure to make exercise part of your weight-loss regime. Exercising for at least half an hour a day will increase the number of calories burned. Refer to the Calories Burned with Exercise chart on page 30 for an idea of how many calories are burned per hour with various types of activities. Adopt healthy eating habits that will enable you to lose weight and to keep it off as well. A weight loss of 1–2 pounds a week is considered reasonable and safe. Adult males tend to lose excess weight faster than adult females. If you experience the so-called dieter's plateau—a stretch of time during which there is very little or no weight loss despite adherence to an eating and exercise plan—be patient. This slowdown happens to almost everyone and is usually temporary. Adhere to a program of healthy eating and exercise and your goal will be reached. Consult the chart on page 219 to determine ideal weight. One question often asked is, "How many calories do I need to eat per day to lose weight?"

This depends upon a person's age, body size, and level of physical activity. To lose one pound of weight per week, a person needs to trim 500 calories a day (3,500 calories a week) from the amount currently being eaten or 1,000 calories a day (7,000 a week) to lose 2 pounds a week. To understand better where the calories are coming from, keep track of what is eaten for several typical days, using the Food Diary (page 220). Then, begin to alter food selections, preparation methods, and/or portion sizes to deduct the necessary calories. To define more closely calorie needs for weight loss, use the worksheet on page 222. A diet consisting of fewer than 1,200 calories a day is not recommended unless it is supervised by a health care provider.

Two restricted-calorie diets with 7-day menu plans for each appear on the following pages. Generally, the 1,200-calorie plan is appropriate for individuals who are less active or when a faster weight loss (2 pounds a week) is desired, while the 1,800-calorie diet is more suitable for slower weight loss (one pound a week) or for more active persons.

Calculating Your Calorie Quota

The following is a method for estimating roughly the calorie needs for healthy, nonpregnant adults, ages 18–50 years. Older individuals should further reduce calories by 10% to 20%.

A. Refer to the chart on page 219 and determine a realistic ideal weight in the range shown for your height.

Generally, the higher weights in the range apply to men, who usually have more muscle and bone mass than most women. The lower weights in the range more often apply to women.

IDEAL WEIGHT _____ pounds

B. Classify yourself by lifestyle.

_____ Less Active   Little or no regular exercise, desk job

_____ Active   Moderate level of regular exercise, active at work

_____ Very Active   Strenuous regular exercise, manual labor at work

C. Determine your energy need by multiplying your Ideal Weight by your activity level:

      Less Active = 13   Active = 15   Very Active = 17

_____ × _____ = _____ Calories a day

(This is the level of calories that will be needed for weight maintenance once your goal weight is achieved.)

D. Subtract calories for weight loss.

_____ − 500 = _____ Calories a day to lose 1 pound a week
(Calories from
section C)

_____ − 1000 = _____ Calories a day to lose 2 pounds a week
(Calories from
section C)

Note: The lowest recommended calorie intake is 1,200 calories a day for women and 1,500 calories a day for men, even if it would slow down the rate of weight loss. Diets of fewer than 1,200 calories a day tend to be nutritionally inadequate and not effective for long-term weight loss.

DAILY CALORIE GOAL = _____

Calories Burned with Exercise

Weight loss is best accomplished by a sensible reduced-calorie diet and exercise. It takes a deficit of 3,500 calories per week, accomplished by eating less and/or exercising more, to lose one pound. The amount of calories burned depends upon several factors including body size, body composition, age, gender, and the intensity of the exercise performed. The chart below gives a general idea of the amount of calories burned per hour during various activities. Most women should use the values at the lower end of the range, while the upper range is usually appropriate for men.

Activity	Calories Burned per hour
Aerobics, light	345–445
Aerobics, moderate	425–550
Aerobics, step, moderate	625–825
Baseball	275–350
Basketball, easy game	400–500
Biking/cycling, 6 m.p.h.	250–325
Cleaning	175–250
Dancing	325–425
Gardening, moderate	275–375

Golf, walking with bag	400–500
Hiking, moderate	275–375
Jogging/running, 10-min. mile	575–750
Jogging/running, 6-min. mile	900–1200
Laundry	175–250
Mowing, self-propelled mower	200–275
Nordic track, moderate	525–700
Racquetball, moderate	550–725
Shopping	200–275
Shoveling snow	375–475
Skiing, downhill	375–475
Stairmaster, 60 steps/min.	400–500
Swimming, moderate	325–450
Tennis, moderate	375–475
Walking, 20-min. mile	175–250
Walking, 15-min. mile	225–300

Values derived from the Food Processor Plus Nutrition Analysis Systems, ESHA Research, Salem, Oregon.
Reference subjects: 40-year-old woman, 5'5" tall, 140 pounds; 40-year-old man, 5'11" tall, 180 pounds. You may burn more calories if you are younger, taller, or heavier than reference subjects and fewer calories if you are shorter, older, or lighter than reference subjects.

7-DAY MENU PLAN: 1,200 Calories

Note: All margarine is tub form from corn oil. Oils used in food preparation are preferably canola, olive, or corn. The portion sizes listed for meat, fish, poultry, rice, stuffing, pasta, hot cereal, and hot vegetables are based upon weight or cup measurement *after* cooking. Beverages such as plain coffee or tea, water, or sugar-free soft drinks have a negligible nutritional value and can be used freely. Be sure to count the calories of other fluids such as regular soda, punch, or juice.

Diets of 1,200 calories or less tend to be low in calcium and fiber if not carefully planned. Use high-fiber bread and grain products and calcium-fortified foods (some cereals, juices, and breads) whenever possible.

SUNDAY
Breakfast
2 buckwheat pancakes, grilled using about 1 tsp. canola oil and 2 Tbsp. maple syrup, and topped with 1 tsp. soft tub margarine
1 cup 1% fat milk

Lunch
- 1½ cups mixed green salad with ¼ cup chickpeas and 1 Tbsp. vinaigrette
- 1 whole wheat dinner roll
- 1 large orange

Dinner
- 2 oz. roasted or grilled chicken breast, no skin
- ¾ cup steamed asparagus
- ¾ cup wild rice
- 1 tsp. soft tub margarine

Snacks and Treats
- 1 cup low-fat fruit yogurt

MONDAY
Breakfast
- 1 whole wheat bagel
- 1 tsp. soft tub margarine
- 2 Tbsp. jam
- 1 cup 1% fat milk

Lunch
- ½ tuna salad sandwich:
  - 1 oz. canned light tuna, packed in water, mixed with 1 Tbsp. mayonnaise
  - Lettuce and tomato
  - 1 slice pumpernickel bread
- ¼ cup dried apricots

Dinner
- 2 oz. roast pork, trimmed
- ½ cup unsweetened applesauce
- ¾ cup steamed broccoli
- ½ cup steamed corn

Snacks and Treats
- 1 cup low-fat fruit yogurt

TUESDAY
Breakfast
- ½ medium grapefruit
- 1 small bran muffin
- 1 cup 1% fat milk

Lunch
- ½ turkey sandwich:
    - 1 oz. turkey breast
    - Lettuce and tomato
    - 2 tsp. honey mustard
    - 1 slice whole wheat bread
- 1 small apple

Dinner
- 1½ cup mixed green salad with 1 Tbsp. vinaigrette dressing
- Spaghetti with meatballs:
    - 1 cup cooked spaghetti noodles
    - 2 meatballs (about 1½ oz. extra-lean ground beef)
    - ½ cup marinara sauce
- 1 Tbsp. low-sodium Parmesan cheese

Snacks and Treats
- 1 cup low-fat fruit yogurt
- ¼ oz. sunflower seeds

WEDNESDAY
Breakfast
- 1 whole wheat English muffin
- 1 Tbsp. jam
- 1 cup 1% fat milk

Lunch
- Chef's salad:
    - 1 cup mixed greens
    - 1 oz. turkey breast
    - 1 oz. low-sodium Swiss cheese
    - 1 Tbsp. Italian dressing
- 15 grapes

Dinner

Tofu stir-fry:
- 2 tsp. canola oil
- ½ cup tofu (about 4 oz.)
- ½ cup mixed vegetables, such as pea pods, carrots, and mushrooms
- 1 Tbsp. reduced sodium soy sauce
- 1 cup brown rice
- ½ cup pineapple slices

Snacks and Treats

- 1 cup 1% fat milk
- 4 gingersnap cookies

THURSDAY
Breakfast

- 1 cup oatmeal
- 1 tsp. soft tub margarine
- 1 Tbsp. honey
- ½ banana
- 1 cup 1% fat milk

Lunch

½ roast beef sandwich:
- 1 oz. roast beef
- Lettuce
- 2 tsp. mustard
- 1 slice rye bread
- ½ cup honeydew melon

Dinner

Turkey chili:
- 2 oz. ground turkey
- ½ cup kidney or pinto beans
- 1 cup low-sodium diced tomatoes
- ½ cup barley
- 1 Tbsp. shredded low-sodium cheddar cheese

Snacks and Treats

- 1 cup low-fat fruit yogurt

FRIDAY
Breakfast
- 1 cup bran flake cereal
- ½ cup blueberries
- 1 cup 1% fat milk

Lunch
- 1 cup lentil soup
- 1 slice multigrain bread
- ½ cup tomato and cucumber salad with vinaigrette dressing
- 1 medium pear

Dinner
- 2 oz. baked or broiled trout
- ½ baked sweet potato
- 1 tsp. soft tub margarine
- 1 cup stir-fried green beans with almonds (1 Tbsp. chopped blanched almonds, 1 tsp. olive oil)

Snacks and Treats
- 1 cup 1% fat milk
- 2 graham cracker squares

SATURDAY
Breakfast
- Mushroom, onion, and pepper egg-white omelet, prepared with 1 tsp. canola oil, 1% fat milk, and 4 egg whites
- ½ cup cantaloupe
- 1 cup 1% fat milk

Lunch
- Chicken vegetable stew:
  - 1 oz. stewed chicken
  - 1 cup mixed vegetables (carrots, green beans, corn, onions, celery)
  - 1 cup whole wheat noodles

Dinner
- 1 cup tossed salad with 1 tsp. balsamic vinegar and 1 tsp. olive oil
- 1 slice cheese pizza

Snacks and Treats
- 2 plums

7-DAY MENU PLAN: 1,800 Calories

Note: Optional: Plain coffee or tea, water, dietetic beverages. Be sure to count the calories of other beverages such as regular soft drinks, punch, or juice. All margarine is from corn oil. Fats allotted for food preparation are included in the meal plan. Otherwise, use non-stick cooking spray. The portion sizes listed for meat, poultry, fish, rice, stuffing, pasta, hot cereal, and hot vegetables are based upon weight or cup measurements *after* cooking.

SUNDAY
Breakfast
2 buckwheat pancakes, grilled using about 1 tsp. canola oil and
    topped with 1 tsp. tub margarine and 2 Tbsp. maple syrup
½ cup fresh fruit salad
1 cup 1% fat milk

Lunch
Hamburger:
    3 oz. extra-lean ground beef, broiled
    1 Tbsp. catsup
    Lettuce and tomato
    Whole wheat bun
10 oven-baked steak fries with 1 Tbsp. catsup
1 cup low-fat fruit yogurt

Dinner
2½ oz. roasted or grilled chicken breast, no skin
1 cup steamed asparagus
1 cup wild rice
1 large orange

Snacks and Treats
1 cup 1% fat milk
2 graham cracker squares

MONDAY
Breakfast
1 whole wheat bagel
1 Tbsp. peanut butter
1 cup 1% fat milk

Lunch
> Tuna salad sandwich:
>> 2 oz. canned light tuna, packed in water, with celery and 1 Tbsp. mayonnaise
>>
>> Lettuce and tomato
>>
>> 2 slices pumpernickel bread
>
> 1 cup low-fat fruit yogurt
>
> 1 large peach

Dinner
> 2 oz. roast pork, trimmed
>
> ⅓ cup unsweetened applesauce
>
> 1 cup steamed broccoli
>
> 1 medium baked potato
>
> 2 tsp. tub margarine

Snacks and Treats
> 1 cup 1% fat milk
>
> 4 fig bar cookies

TUESDAY
Breakfast
> ½ grapefruit
>
> 1 bran muffin
>
> 1 Tbsp. jam
>
> 1 cup 1% fat milk

Lunch
> Turkey sandwich:
>> 2 oz. turkey breast
>>
>> Lettuce and tomato
>>
>> 2 tsp. honey mustard
>>
>> 2 slices whole wheat bread
>
> ½ cup baby carrots
>
> 1 small apple

Dinner
> 2 cups mixed green salad with 2 Tbsp. vinaigrette dressing
>
> Spaghetti with meatballs:
>> 1½ cups cooked spaghetti noodles

2 meatballs (about 2 oz. extra-lean ground beef)
¾ cup marinara sauce
2 Tbsp. low-sodium Parmesan cheese

Snacks and Treats
1 cup low-fat fruit yogurt
½ oz. sunflower seeds, hulled

WEDNESDAY
Breakfast
1 whole wheat English muffin
1 Tbsp. jam
1 scrambled egg, using about 1 tsp. tub margarine and
   1% fat milk
1 cup 1% fat milk

Lunch
Chef's salad:
   2 cups mixed greens
   1 medium tomato, quartered
   1½ oz. turkey
   1 oz. low-sodium Swiss cheese
   2 Tbsp. Italian dressing
4 sesame bread sticks
15 grapes

Dinner
Tofu stir-fry:
   2 tsp. canola oil
   ¾ cup tofu (about 6 oz.)
   1½ cup mixed vegetables such as pea pods, carrots, bean
      sprouts, mushrooms, broccoli baby corn, water chestnuts
   2 Tbsp. reduced-sodium soy sauce
1 cup brown rice
1 cup pineapple slices in own juice

Snacks and Treats
1 cup 1% fat milk
4 gingersnap cookies

THURSDAY
Breakfast
- 1 cup oatmeal
- 1 Tbsp. honey
- 1 large banana
- 1 cup 1% fat milk

Lunch
Roast beef sandwich:
- 2 oz. roast beef
- Lettuce and tomato
- 2 tsp. mustard
- 2 slices rye bread
- 1 cup coleslaw
- ½ cup honeydew melon

Dinner
Turkey chili:
- 2 oz. ground turkey
- ½ cup kidney or pinto beans
- ½ cup low-sodium diced tomatoes
- ½ cup barley
- ¼ cup shredded low-sodium cheddar cheese
- 1 small piece of cornbread

Snacks and Treats
- 1 cup low-fat fruit yogurt

FRIDAY
Breakfast
- 1 cup bran flake cereal
- ½ cup blueberries
- 1 cup 1% fat milk

Lunch
- 1 bowl lentil soup
- 2 slices multigrain bread
- 2 oz. low-sodium Swiss cheese
- 1 cup tomato and cucumber salad with vinaigrette dressing
- 1 medium pear

Dinner

- 3 oz. baked or broiled trout
- 1 large baked sweet potato
- 1 cup stir-fried green beans with almonds (1 Tbsp. chopped blanched almonds, 1 tsp. olive oil)

Snacks and Treats

- 1 slice angel food cake with ½ cup strawberries
- 1 cup fat-free frozen yogurt

SATURDAY

Breakfast

- Mushroom, onion, and pepper egg-white omelet, prepared with 1 tsp. canola oil and 4 egg whites
- 2 slices whole wheat toast
- 2 tsp. tub margarine
- 1 cup cantaloupe
- 1 cup 1% fat milk

Lunch

- Chicken vegetable stew:
  - 3 oz. stewed chicken
  - 1 cup mixed vegetables (carrots, green beans, corn, potatoes, onions, celery)
- 1 cup whole wheat noodles
- 1 cup low-fat fruit yogurt

Dinner

- 2 cups tossed salad with 2 Tbsp. vinaigrette dressing
- 2 slices cheese pizza from large pie

Snacks and Treats

- 2 plums

SPECIAL DIETS

Low-Sodium Diet

Sodium is a mineral that plays a major role in regulating fluid balance in the body. An excessive sodium intake can increase the risk of developing high blood pressure and can further increase blood pressure in individuals with known hypertension. A low-sodium diet is recommended for individuals with certain kidney, heart, and liver disorders and when some medications may interfere with normal fluid balance. Even for healthy individuals, moderation in sodium intake is recommended.

The National Academy of Sciences recommends an average daily intake of no more than 2,400 mg (approx. 1 tsp. salt) of sodium a day for healthy people. Sodium can be further restricted in the treatment of particular medical conditions such as uncontrolled hypertension, congestive heart failure, and liver and kidney diseases associated with fluid retention. The minimum amount of sodium needed for health is 500 mg a day, or the amount in ¼ teaspoon of table salt. Most Americans take in far more sodium than is necessary or desirable.

The major source of sodium in the typical American diet is table salt (sodium chloride) that is used in food preparation, at the table, and in the manufacture of processed, prepared, and convenience food items. The food industry has developed many low- and reduced-sodium products that are widely available. Refer to the section Reading Food Labels (page 9) for more information. While sodium does occur naturally in most foods, the amount is usually small. In general, diets are lowest in sodium when very little processed, prepared, and convenience foods are used and when whole grains, fresh fruits, vegetables, and meat, fish, and poultry (all prepared without salt) are emphasized.

GENERAL GUIDELINES:

1. Omit or reduce the use of table salt, salt-based spices, and high-sodium condiments. Use more herbs, spices, lemon juice, or herbal vinegars for flavor. Only use salt substitutes with permission of your physician as they contain more potassium than is desirable for some people.

2. Buy as many fresh foods as possible, and limit the use of processed, prepared, and convenience foods.

3. When canned, frozen, or packaged foods are purchased, check the labels to identify the sodium content per serving of that item. Avoid purchasing items with claims such as "reduced sodium" or "light in

sodium" and, instead, identify the milligrams of sodium per serving. Foods that contain more than 480 mg of sodium per serving should be used less frequently.

4. Refer to the list of foods below, which are typically significant sources of sodium. Foods not appearing on the list contain some natural sodium but not in high quantities.

Foods to Limit or Avoid

Bread, Cereal, Rice, and Pasta
Cake mixes (especially angel food and chocolate; check labels)
Cereals (some dry and instant hot varieties; check labels)
Cornbread, commercially prepared or from mix
Mixes for biscuits and pancakes, especially buttermilk-type
Macaroni, rice, and stuffing mixes
Prepared frozen macaroni and cheese, pancakes and waffles
Salted crackers
Salted snack foods (cheese curls, popcorn, potato chips, pretzels, snack mixes, tortilla chips)
Seasoned bread crumbs and croutons

Fruits
Maraschino cherries
Some dried fruits (check labels)

Vegetables
Brine-cured (sauerkraut, olives) and marinated (artichoke hearts) vegetables
Canned, unless without added salt
Frozen with sauce
Pickled (pickled beets, pickles, three-bean salad)
Potato mixes, including instant potato flakes
Spaghetti sauce and canned tomato products

Milk, Yogurt, and Cheese
Buttermilk
Cheeses (including Parmesan; reduced- or low-sodium types are available; check labels)
Cheese sauces and spreads
Malted milk and malted-milk drink mixes
Pudding, instant mix

Meat, Poultry, Fish, Eggs, and Nuts
Bacon
Beans (baked beans, canned—unless well rinsed, pork and beans)
Canned items (including anchovies, chicken, chili, chipped beef, chow
  mein, corned beef and corned beef hash, ham and deviled ham, meat
  spreads, salmon, sardines, seafood, stews, tuna)
Fast foods
Frankfurters (except low-sodium types)
Frozen TV dinners, entrees, fish fillets, fried or breaded chicken (most)
Kielbasa
Luncheon meats (most, except "low-sodium" varieties)
Nuts, if salted
Pizza
Sausage
Smoked fish, meats, and poultry

Fats, Oils, and Sweets
Gravy mixes
Salad dressing (most)
Salt pork

Miscellaneous
Bacon bits
Barbecue sauce
Catsup (unless low-sodium; use regular types very sparingly)
Meat tenderizers
Monosodium glutamate (MSG)
Prepared mustard (use very sparingly)
Relish
Salsa
Salt, including "lite" types and salt-based spices such as garlic salt,
  onion salt, and seasoned salt; read labels on spice mixes as there may
  be hidden sodium (some lemon-pepper spices)
Sauce mix packages and bottled sauces
Steak sauce
Soups and broth (canned, condensed, cubes, dehydrated; some reduced-
  or low-sodium varieties acceptable)
Soy sauce, including "lite" types
Tartar sauce
Teriyaki sauce

Heart Healthy Eating

Most Americans eat too much fat, saturated fat, and cholesterol, which are major factors in the development of heart disease. High blood cholesterol levels can often be treated by a diet containing lesser amounts of these nutrients.

A type of cholesterol called low density lipoprotein, or "LDL," can promote atherosclerosis or plaque buildup in the arteries that supply blood to the heart. However, high density lipoprotein, or "HDL," another type of cholesterol, is protective against heart disease. A diet that is too high in saturated fat and cholesterol can increase LDL cholesterol levels. Smoking, obesity, and lack of physical activity can lower HDL cholesterol levels. All adults should have their blood cholesterol level checked by their physician.

GUIDELINES FOR IMPLEMENTATION

1. The calories in your diet should be appropriate for achieving and maintaining your ideal weight (see Suggested Weights for Adults, p. 219, and Calculating Your Calorie Quota, p. 29). Being too fat, especially if you are apple-shaped (waist circumference more than 40″ for men, more than 35″ for women), can increase risk of heart disease.

2. Obtain 20%–35% of your calories from total fat. To calculate fat requirements, first determine overall calorie needs. By multiplying calorie needs by 0.20 and by 0.35, the daily diet range of fat calories can be determined. Then divide the upper and lower values of fat calories by 9, the number of calories per gram of fat. This will result in recommended fat grams allowed per day.

   EXAMPLE: 1,800 calories × 0.20 = 360 fat calories; × 0.35 = 630 fat calories.
   360 fat calories ÷ 9 = 40 grams of fat; 630 fat calories ÷ 9 = 70 grams of fat.

3. About 10% of daily calories or less should be from saturated fat. This is the type of fat found in animal products as well as solid vegetable fats and tropical oils.

   EXAMPLE: 1,800 calories × 0.10 = 180 saturated fat calories
   180 saturated fat calories ÷ 9 = 20 grams of saturated fat

Replace saturated fats with unsaturated sources. Polyunsaturated fats include safflower, soybean, sunflower, and corn oil, and margarine made with these oils. Avoid using hydrogenated sources such as sticks of margarine, vegetable shortening, and products prepared with hydrogenated vegetable oil as the first type of fat in the list of ingredients. Hydrogenation appears to increase the amount of another undesirable fat called trans fat. Monounsaturated fats are olive, peanut, and canola oils. Overall, monounsaturated fats are preferable but should still be used as part of the total fat allowance.

4. Limit dietary cholesterol, which is found only in animal foods, to 300 mg a day. Accomplish this by choosing up to 6½ oz. equivalents of lean sources from the meat and beans group per day and by limiting eggs, shellfish, and organ meats.

5. Take in adequate amounts of fiber, particularly soluble fiber as found in beans, lentils, fresh fruits, oats, and barley.

6. If following the above guidelines does not optimize your blood cholesterol levels, reduce dietary cholesterol intake to 200 mg a day and saturated fat to 7% or less of daily calories. At this point, seek the assistance of a registered dietitian.

7. Individuals with a high level of triglycerides (a type of blood fat) should avoid alcoholic beverages and limit high-sugar foods in addition to the above.

Many experts feel that further reducing total fat intake to as low as 10% of daily calories is appropriate. This may be effective for some types of cholesterol elevations but not all. Very low-fat, high-carbohydrate diets may further increase elevated triglycerides in some people. Be sure to check with your physician before making drastic dietary changes.

MEAL PLANNING TIPS

1. Many foods from the bread, rice, cereal, and pasta group are very low in fat content (0–1 gram of fat per serving). Focus on choices highest in fiber. Limit the use of snack foods and bakery goods, as they contain a considerable amount of fat. Be sure to count the fats used in preparing these foods. As a spread on top of breads, try jam. Reduced-fat soft margarine and sour cream can be used on top of vegetables or potatoes. Fat-free baked goods are acceptable, but be careful as they often have a high calorie count.

2. Fruits and vegetables by nature contain virtually no fat, saturated fat, or cholesterol. Enhance vegetables by using lemon juice, herbal vinegar, or reduced-fat and fat-free salad dressing. If vegetables are stir-fried, use only a small amount of an acceptable oil or non-stick cooking spray.

3. Dairy products should be low-fat. Look for skim or 1% fat milk, low-fat yogurt, and cheese with fewer than 3 grams of fat per ounce.

4. Choose fish and skinless chicken more often than red meat. When using red meat, buy lean cuts such as extra-lean ground beef, top round, sirloin steak, flank steak, eye round, center, loin or tenderloin pork, leg of lamb, or shoulder lamb chops. Shellfish can be used occasionally, but limit the frequency due to its relatively high cholesterol content. Many luncheon meats, hot dogs, and sausage products are available with an acceptable fat content (read labels to find products that contain fewer than 3 grams of fat per ounce or 10 grams of fat per 3-ounce portion).

   Limit egg yolks to about 3 per week, including what has been used in food preparation. Use egg substitutes or replace one whole egg with two egg whites. Use organ meats infrequently.

   Trim off all visible fat from these foods before preparing them, and use methods such as baking, broiling, roasting, poaching, or grilling as they do not require extra added fat. Above all, keep portion sizes to no more than 6½ ounces daily.

   Some meat alternatives, such as dry beans and peas, contain no fat, saturated fat, or cholesterol. Try to incorporate some "vegetarian" entrees into your diet, such as meatless chili or lentil soup.

5. All added fats should be used in moderation, including unsaturated sources. Regular tub margarine, mayonnaise, and vegetable oils contain about 5 grams of fat per teaspoon, so using them liberally may bankrupt your fat budget quickly. Reduced-fat or "diet" margarine and mayonnaise contain about 5 grams of fat per 1 tablespoon portion. Use more herbs and spices to enhance food flavors. Added fats can often be reduced in quantity or even eliminated entirely.

6. Use alcohol in moderation. Certain alcoholic beverages, such as red wine, may be beneficial for preventing heart disease in some people since it appears to raise protective HDL cholesterol. Remember that alcohol can be a source of excess calories and can interact with many

medications. People with high triglyceride levels may make this condition worse by drinking alcohol.

High-Fiber Diet

Fiber, also known as roughage, is the undigestible portion of plant foods. Fiber helps with proper functioning of the intestinal tract as it speeds the elimination of waste products. A high-fiber diet alleviates constipation and may lower risk of colon cancer. Other intestinal ailments such as diverticular disease, hemorrhoids, and irritable bowel can be prevented and/or treated with a high-fiber diet.

Individuals with diabetes may also benefit from a high-fiber diet since it may improve blood sugar control. Soluble fiber, a type of fiber found in oats, legumes, barley, and some fruits, may help reduce blood cholesterol levels. On a weight-loss diet, fiber may improve success as high-fiber foods (especially vegetables and fruits) tend to be low in calorie content, take a long time to chew, and are quite filling. Most authorities recommend 20–35 grams of fiber daily (some say up to 40 grams a day), but most Americans eat far less. Milk and dairy products, meat, fish and shellfish, poultry, eggs, and fats have an insignificant amount of fiber. Fiber is not broken down as a result of cooking foods.

GUIDELINES FOR IMPLEMENTATION

1. Increase the fiber in the diet slowly to prevent abdominal bloating, gas, and flatulence.

2. Soak beans or lentils overnight in water and rinse well to reduce their gassiness and lessen cooking time.

3. Wash fruits and vegetables well. Try not to remove the skin or peel whenever possible as this usually reduces the fiber content. Choose fresh or even canned fruits over juice.

4. Fiber should be obtained from a variety of whole grains, breads and cereals, fruits, and vegetables. Take a fiber supplement only if recommended by a physician.

5. Fruits and vegetables with small seeds (berries, figs, tomatoes) as well as poppy or sesame seeds should be used with caution by individuals with a history of diverticular disease.

6. Drink an adequate amount of fluids; otherwise, a high-fiber diet may be constipating. Aim for 8 glasses a day.

7. Read food labels to compare the grams of fiber per serving among similar food items, choosing those with the highest fiber content. Use refined grains less frequently.

8. Refer to the list below for more information on the fiber content of various foods.

Fiber Content of Various Foods

6+ grams of fiber per serving

Bread, Cereal, Rice, Pasta, and Meat Alternatives

Beans, cooked (½ cup): baked, black, chickpeas, great northern, kidney, lima, navy, pinto, refried, white
Bean soups (1 cup)
Cold cereals (⅓ cup): 100% Bran, All Bran, Bran Buds, Fiber One
Lentils (½ cup)
Split peas (½ cup)

Vegetables

Artichokes (1 globe)

Fruits

Blackberries (1 cup)
Dried figs, dates (½ cup)
Prunes, stewed (½ cup)
Raspberries (1 cup)

4.1–6.0 grams of fiber per serving

Bread, Cereal, Rice, Pasta, and Meat Alternatives

Beans, cooked (½ cup): soy
Cold cereals (¾ cup): Bran Chex, Bran Flakes, Heartwise, Raisin Bran
Crackers: rye wafers (2)
Grains, cooked (½ cup): barley, buckwheat, bulgur wheat, corn meal, couscous
Green peas, cow peas (½ cup)
Oatmeal, cooked (½ cup)
Oat bran, raw (½ cup)
Whole wheat English muffin (1)

Fruits
Asian pear (1)
Mango (1)
Papaya (1)
Pear (1)

Vegetables
Baby lima beans, cooked (½ cup)

3.1–4.0 grams of fiber per serving
Bread, Cereal, Rice, Pasta, and Meat Alternatives
Bran or oat bran muffin (1)
Cold cereals: Grapenuts (⅓ cup), Shredded Wheat (⅔ cup)
Hummus (¼ cup)
Nuts (1 oz.): almonds
Wheat germ (¼ cup)
Whole wheat pita bread (1)

Fruits
Apple (1)
Banana (1)
Blueberries (1 cup)
Figs, fresh or dried (2)
Orange (1)
Papaya (1 cup)
Stewed prunes (½ cup)
Strawberries (1 cup)

Vegetables
Brussels sprouts, cooked (½ cup)
Mixed vegetables, cooked (½ cup)
Peas, cooked (½ cup)
Pumpkin (½ cup)
Spinach (½ cup)
Sweet potato, without skin (1); baked potato, with skin (1)

2.0–3.0 grams of fiber per serving
Bread, Cereal, Rice, Pasta, and Meat Alternatives
Cold cereals (¾ cup): Cheerios, Oat Flakes, Wheat Chex, Wheaties
Grains (½ cup), buckwheat groats (kasha), couscous

Instant oatmeal (½ cup)
Nuts (1 oz.): hazelnuts, peanuts, pecans, pistachio, macadamia
Oat bran, cooked (½ cup)
Popcorn (3 cups)
Peanut butter, chunky (2 Tbsp.)
Sunflower seeds, dry roasted (¼ cup)
Whole wheat and mixed-grain breads (1 slice) (check labels as fiber content varies)

Fruits
Coconut, dried, flaked (¼ cup)
Guava (1)
Orange (1)
Pears, canned (½ cup); fresh (1)
Raisins (½ cup)
Rhubarb (½ cup)

Vegetables
Broccoli, cooked (½ cup)
Carrots, cooked (½ cup)
Collard greens, cooked (½ cup)
Corn, canned or frozen (½ cup); fresh (1 ear)
Okra (½ cup)
Parsnips, cooked (½ cup)
Pea pods/snow peas (½ cup)
Sauerkraut (½ cup)
Spinach, cooked (¾ cup)
Tomato sauce (⅔ cup)
Turnip greens (½ cup
Winter squash (½ cup)

Foods with less than 2.0 grams of fiber per serving are listed under the Low-Fiber Diet. These foods can also be included in your diet, but unless eaten in great quantity, they will not provide adequate fiber.

Food Ideas:
- Add cooked beans to soups, stews, and casseroles or on top of salads.

- Substitute whole wheat and rye flour in place of all-purpose flour, brown rice for white rice, and spinach or whole wheat pasta for standard pasta.

- Incorporate bran or rolled oats in such main dishes as meatloaf or casseroles.

- Sprinkle a high-fiber cereal on top of your favorite breakfast cereal, mix it into yogurt, or use as topping on frozen desserts.

- Use fruits as snacks and dessert and even try a main dish that incorporates fruit, such as pineapple and chicken.

- Add vegetables to main dishes, casseroles, soups, and stews.

Diabetic Diet

A healthy diet for people with diabetes is very similar to the Dietary Guidelines for Americans. Foods high in fiber and naturally low in fat should be emphasized, such as whole grains, fresh fruits, and vegetables. Dairy products should be low-fat, while meat and meat alternative selections should focus on lean sources with about 5–6½ equivalents total per day. Added fats and sugars should be used sparingly. Calories should be consumed to attain a healthy weight. Protein should comprise about 10–20% of daily calories, fats about 30% of daily calories. Due to increased heart-disease risk associated with diabetes, the American Diabetes Association (ADA) recommends limiting saturated fat to less than 7% of total calories, dietary cholesterol to less than 200 mg per day, and minimizing intake of trans fat. Finally, about 50% of daily calories should come from carbohydrates. The exact breakdown of calories can vary, depending upon blood glucose levels and the presence of other medical conditions such as a high blood cholesterol or triglyceride level.

    For nearly a century, people with diabetes were told to avoid simple carbohydrates (such as table sugar, maple syrup, and corn syrup) because they dramatically increase blood glucose levels. Instead, starches or complex carbohydrates (such as bread, rice, potatoes, cereals, and pastas) were encouraged. Recent guidelines do not strictly prohibit the use of simple carbohydrates because there is insufficient proof that they raise blood sugar any more than starches. Instead, as with everyone, sugar in all its forms should be used in moderation. It is now recommended that the diabetic diet focus on the total amount of carbohydrate (about 50% of daily calories) as opposed to the form of carbohydrate obtained. If sugars are used, they should be counted as part of the carbohydrate allowed each day and not just an extra item added into the diet.

Because foods high in sugar are often high in calories and provide few vitamins and minerals, they should not be overused.

Individuals with insulin-dependent diabetes (type I) need to pay close attention to consistency in meal and snack composition, size, and times of day to keep blood sugar as near normal levels as possible. Additional planning is needed to avoid and treat hypoglycemia, especially when one is sick or has exercised more than usual.

Those with non-insulin-dependent diabetes (type II) often need to focus on reaching a healthy weight, getting more exercise, and, like all Americans, eating less fat, saturated fat, cholesterol, sodium, and sugar. A weight loss of 10–20 pounds can improve blood glucose levels for many people.

In summary, there is no longer any one "correct" diabetic diet. In addition to the Dietary Guidelines for Americans, other strategies for a healthy diabetic diet include using the Exchange Lists for Meal Planning by the American Diabetes Association and the American Dietetic Association and counting carbohydrate grams. A registered dietitian (R.D.) can help develop a meal plan that is best suited for an individual's needs and includes the foods the individual enjoys eating, even some sugary foods on occasion. For more information, contact the American Diabetes Association at 1-800-232-6733. The Nutrition Consumer Hotline at the National Center for Nutrition and Dietetics, 1-800-366-1655, can help you locate a registered dietitian in your area.

Vegetarian Diet

A vegetarian is someone who excludes one or more types of animal products. There are several types of vegetarians. A lacto-ovo-vegetarian excludes meat, fish, poultry, and seafood but does include milk, milk products, and eggs. A lacto-vegetarian will further exclude eggs, while a vegan only eats plant foods. Semi-vegetarians usually consume some type of fish or poultry but do not eat red meats.

Since vegetarian diets focus on plant-based foods, they have the potential to be lower in fat, saturated fat, and cholesterol and higher in fiber content than the typical American diet. Except for a vegan diet, the other vegetarian diets can be nutritionally adequate if wisely chosen. Vegans need to supplement vitamin B12 (found only in animal foods) or consistently include foods fortified with this nutrient, such as many

soybean products. Calcium, zinc, iron, vitamin D (depending on sunlight exposure), and riboflavin may also be low in this very restrictive
diet.

Diets that include eggs and/or milk and milk products will provide
high-quality protein in which all essential amino acids should be present.
Plant foods contain protein, but usually of lower quality because one or
more essential amino acids is lacking or low.

GUIDELINES FOR IMPLEMENTATION

1. Generally speaking, it is recommended that foods from the bread,
   rice, and pasta group be combined with either vegetables, legumes,
   or nuts or seeds (meat alternatives) to ensure that the amino acids
   naturally low in this group are obtained. Soy protein is considered to
   be equal in quality to animal protein. However, it is no longer considered critical to have certain combinations or "complementary"
   proteins in the same meal, but rather to focus on a variety of foods
   from each group over the entire day. Meal suggestions using plant
   foods include:

Sautéed vegetables with brown rice	Couscous with vegetables
Rice or pasta and beans	Hummus on pita bread
Lentil soup with peanut butter crackers	Vegetable salad topped with nuts/seeds
Vegetarian chili with cornbread	Stir-fried tofu with vegetables over rice

2. Pay careful attention to the nutrients that may be lacking in a diet,
   based upon which foods are excluded, and use nutritional supplements as appropriate.

3. Adapt the food groups below for meal planning based upon individual preferences:

Foods Allowed

Bread, Cereal, Rice, and Pasta
Whole grain bread, cereals, rice, and pasta
Baked goods prepared without animal fat

Fruits and Vegetables
All, including texturized vegetable protein products

Meat Alternatives
Eggs (for lacto-ovo-vegetarians)
Nuts, peanut butter, seeds
Legumes (cooked dry beans, peas, lentils, peanuts)
Tofu (soybean curd)
Milk and Milk Products
All (for lacto- and lacto-ovo-vegetarians)
Soy milk

Fats and Sugars
Vegetable oil, vegetable shortening, soft tub margarine
Sugar, jam, jelly, honey, corn syrup

Lactose-Restricted Diet

Many people are not able to fully digest lactose, the type of sugar found in milk and milk products, due to a deficiency of an enzyme called lactase. Symptoms of lactose intolerance include abdominal bloating, stomach cramps, and diarrhea. Consult a doctor if lactose intolerance is suspected.

GUIDELINES FOR IMPLEMENTATION

1. Tailor the diet to meet a personal level of tolerance for lactose. Some people can tolerate small amounts of lactose, particularly from fermented milk products such as aged cheeses, yogurt with active cultures, and cottage cheese.

2. Unless adequate calcium is consistently obtained from non-dairy sources, talk with a doctor about taking a calcium supplement.

3. Reduced-lactose dairy products such as milk or cheese are available, but they are usually not completely lactose-free. Lactase enzyme has been added to these products to "predigest" most of the lactose. Use these products if they are tolerated to help create a diet more nutritionally balanced and adequate in calcium. Ask a doctor about the use of over-the-counter lactase enzyme preparations.

4. Always read labels to identify hidden sources of lactose from food processing. Key words to look for include *milk, milk solids, non-fat dry milk, milk powder, whey, curd,* and *lactose.* Avoid foods with these

ingredients. Lactic acid, lactalbumin, and lactate do not contain lactose or milk and can safely be used.

5. Refer to the list below of foods to avoid or strictly limit.

Foods to Avoid

Bread, Cereal, Rice, and Pasta
Any product prepared with milk or milk solids; check label
Some cold and instant hot cereals
Products prepared with butter or milk-containing margarine
Rice and pasta mixes with dehydrated cheese, cream, or milk solids
Baking mixes, including pancake, biscuit, and cookie

Vegetables
Creamed vegetables
Vegetables or potatoes prepared with butter or milk-containing margarine
Frozen vegetables and potatoes if processed with lactose
Instant potato flakes and mixes with dehydrated cheese or cream sauce

Fruits
Canned or frozen if processed with lactose

Meat, Poultry, Fish, Dry Beans and Peas, Eggs, and Nuts
Eggs prepared with milk, cheese, butter, or milk-containing margarine
Cold cuts and hot dogs with milk solids
Creamed or many breaded meat, fish, or poultry items

Milk and Milk Products
Cheese
Cocoa mixes
Ice cream, ice milk, frozen yogurt, sherbet
Custard, mousse, and pudding
Milk, buttermilk, chocolate milk, evaporated milk, malted milk, sweetened condensed milk (some people may be able to use milk treated with lactase)
Yogurt if not tolerated

Fats and Sugars
Butter
Cream and cream sauces

Gravy with butter, milk-containing margarine, cream, or milk solids
Margarine containing milk
Salad dressings containing milk or milk products
Sour cream
Some candies: butterscotch, caramels, chocolate, toffee
Miscellaneous
Soups prepared with milk or cream
Canned soup or dry mixes containing milk or nonfat milk solids

Foods Allowed
(Always check labels)

Bread, Cereal, Rice, and Pasta
Products prepared without butter, milk-containing margarine, milk, or
    milk solids (usually includes hard rolls, French and Italian breads,
    soda crackers, angel food cake)
Cooked plain cereal
Pasta, rice

Vegetables
Plain fresh, canned, or frozen to which no lactose has been added

Fruits
Plain fresh, canned, or frozen to which no lactose has been added

Meat, Poultry, Fish, Dry Beans and Peas, Eggs, and Nuts
Kosher cold cuts and hot dogs
Plain beef, chicken, lamb, organ meats, pork, poultry, veal
Eggs, poached, boiled, or prepared with acceptable ingredients
Peanut butter, nuts, seeds, and cooked dry beans and peas

Milk and Milk Products
Some people may tolerate a small amount of milk products, including
    yogurt and lactase-treated milk and cheese

Fats and Sugars
Milk-free margarine
Many non-dairy creamers
Oils
Salad dressing without milk or milk solids
Vegetable shortening

Fruit ice, sorbet, gelatin
Sugar, jam, jelly, honey, corn syrup, most hard candy

Dietary Guidelines for Gout

The occurrence of gout is associated with a diet that is excessive in purine content. Purines are normally converted into uric acid, which is then eliminated in the urine. In people prone to gout, uric acid levels are often high due to an increased rate of formation of uric acid and to a diminished rate of excretion. When uric acid builds up in the bloodstream, crystals are formed that can then deposit in the joints (big toe, foot, ankle, knee). These deposits cause a painful inflammation and can also be responsible for uric acid kidney stones. It is recommended that individuals with gout avoid an excessive purine intake so that less uric acid is produced.

Much of the purines in the typical American diet are obtained from animal proteins such as meat, poultry, fish, and shellfish. It is therefore recommended that serving sizes of these foods be kept to about 5–7 ounces daily. The difference in calories can be made up with foods high in carbohydrate, such as breads, grains, fruits, and vegetables. A high-carbohydrate diet actually helps increase the excretion of uric acid. Asparagus, mushrooms, and spinach contain a moderate amount of purine. Cooked dried beans and peas (kidney beans, white beans, chickpeas, black-eyed peas, etc.) and lentils also contain a substantial amount of purine. They can, however, be used in place of meat, fish, or poultry as an alternative source of protein.

The foods highest in purine content to be avoided are:

Anchovies
Bouillon, broth, consommé, and meat-based soups
Goose
Gravy
Herring
Mackerel
Meat-based extracts (used in gravies, sauces, soups, processed foods)
Mincemeat
Mussels
Organ meats, including brains, heart, kidney, liver, pancreas (sweet-
     breads)

Partridge
Roe (fish eggs)
Sardines
Scallops
Yeast

Other nutritional factors such as consuming excessive fat or alcohol, being overweight, and not drinking enough fluid are known to negatively affect uric acid levels. In addition to the above, it is suggested that one attain or maintain an ideal body weight and lose any excess weight slowly (rapid weight loss may increase uric acid levels); keep fat intake to no more than 30% of daily calories; drink alcohol in moderation; and drink 6–8 glasses of water daily.

Diet for Postprandial (Reactive) Hypoglycemia

Reactive hypoglycemia is a condition resulting in a low blood sugar level about 2–5 hours after a meal and then resolving spontaneously. This is different from the hypoglycemia associated with insulin or other medications for diabetes. Characteristics of reactive hypoglycemia include sweating, weakness, feeling faint, anxiety, and hunger. Diagnosis of reactive hypoglycemia can be made only through laboratory testing by a physician.

There is much disagreement about what type of diet is best for reactive hypoglycemia. Often, the appropriate regimen can only be determined on a trial-and-error basis. If a doctor has diagnosed reactive hypoglycemia, try the following suggestions as a start:

1. Attain and maintain your ideal body weight by eating the appropriate number of calories and engaging in regular physical activity.

2. Eat three meals and two to three snacks a day. Be consistent about meal times and do not skip meals or snacks. Meals and snacks should encompass a variety of foods so that a mixture of protein, fat, and carbohydrate is obtained.

3. There is some evidence that foods high in sugar (thus high in total carbohydrate) should be strictly limited. This includes items such as cake, candy, cookies, Danish, doughnuts, honey, maple syrup, pie, sweetened cereal, canned fruits and juices, most frozen desserts, reg-

ular soda, pudding, and gelatin. These foods are probably best tolerated as part of a meal, as opposed to a snack.

4. The carbohydrates chosen should be complex sources such as whole grain breads and cereals, beans or lentils, rice, pasta, or potatoes. Focus on the choices that are highest in fiber content, particularly soluble fiber as found in fresh fruits, beans or lentils, barley, and oats.

5. People vary in the amount of total carbohydrate tolerated. Adjust your diet according to what alleviates your symptoms.

6. It you drink alcohol, do so in moderation. Alcohol is best tolerated as part of a meal.

High-Calcium Diet

The Dietary Reference Intakes (DRIs) for calcium: 1,000 mg of calcium a day for adults ages 19–50; 1,200 mg of calcium a day for ages 51 and higher is recommended. Many scientists believe that this amount of calcium may not be sufficient to prevent osteoporosis, a condition in which bone loss occurs, increasing the risk of bone fractures. In addition to inadequate calcium intake, other controllable lifestyle risk factors for osteoporosis include inadequate exercise, cigarette smoking, lack of other nutrients such as vitamin D, and excessive intake of alcohol and sodium.

At a minimum, be sure to meet the DRI for calcium, preferably from food sources. It appears that taking in even more calcium than the DRI may be beneficial but not to exceed the Tolerable Uptake Limit Level of 2,500 mg per day. If osteoporosis is diagnosed, ask a doctor how much calcium is needed.

Below is a list of foods that are rich in calcium. The portion size listed provides about 300 mg of calcium. To meet the RDA, 3–4 servings a day from this list are needed. To keep calories, fat, and cholesterol intakes in balance, use low-fat dairy products.

Food	Portion Size for 300 mg calcium
Broccoli	3–4 cups
Cheese, natural	1.5 oz.
Cheese, processed	2 oz.
Cottage cheese	2 cups
Ice cream	2 cups

Juice, calcium fortified	1 cup
Milk	1 cup
Pudding	1 cup
Ricotta cheese	½ cup
Salmon, canned with bone	5 oz. (1 cup)
Sardines	3 oz.
Total cereal	¼ cups
Turnip greens	⅔ cups
Yogurt, carton or frozen	1 cup

Read labels to evaluate foods for their calcium content. A food that is a good source of calcium will provide at least 20% daily value for calcium. If a diet cannot be altered to get adequate calcium, discuss the use of calcium supplements with a physician.

Low-Fiber Diet

Physicians sometimes recommend a low-fiber (also called fiber-restricted) diet (less than 20 grams of fiber a day) for individuals with intestinal problems. During the acute phases of Crohn's disease, ulcerative colitis, and diverticulitis, or after intestinal surgery, a low-fiber diet decreases the amount of waste products that need to be eliminated so that the intestinal tract is not aggravated or irritated. In some cases, a low-residue diet is advised, which further limits the use of certain fruits and vegetables as well as any meats with tough connective tissues.

Note that cooking, mashing, or puréeing foods does not change their fiber content. However, cooked (including canned) fruits and vegetables may cause less gas and are often more easily tolerated than raw fruits or vegetables.

GUIDELINES FOR IMPLEMENTATION

1. Whenever possible, use refined grains such as all-purpose flour and white rice.

2. Remove the skin or peel from fruits and vegetables and the tough membranes from meat.

3. Avoid breads and crackers with nuts, bran, poppy, rye, or sesame seeds.

4. Avoid fruit pies and other desserts that may have nuts, coconut, raisins, or small seeds (blueberry pie, pecan pie).

5. Milk and milk products, meat, poultry, fish and shellfish, and fats do not contain fiber. If "residue" should be limited per doctor's orders, use only tender meats and milk products in moderation.

Foods to Limit or Avoid

Refer to the High-Fiber Diet (page 47) for foods higher in fiber content (more than 2.0 grams of fiber per serving) that should be avoided or used in extreme moderation.

Foods Allowed

1.0–2.0 grams of fiber per serving

Bread, Cereal, Rice, Pasta, and Meat Alternatives

Apple pie (1 small slice)
Bagel, plain or egg (1)
Breads (1 slice): French, Italian, white; some rye, oat, and wheat breads (read labels carefully)
Brown rice, cooked (½ cup)
Corn bread (1 piece), corn muffin (1), corn tortilla (1), or tortilla chips (1 oz.)
Dry cereal (¾ cup) (check labels)
English muffin (1)
Hot cereal (1 cup): Cream of Rice, Cream of Wheat
Pasta (½ cup)
Peanut butter, smooth (2 Tbsp.)
Tortilla, flour (1)

Fruits

Applesauce (½ cup)
Apricots, canned halves (½ cup), fresh (2)
Cantaloupe (1 cup), honeydew (1 cup)
Cherries (10)
Fruit cocktail, canned (½ cup)
Grapefruit (½)
Mandarin orange (1 cup)
Peaches, canned (½ cup), fresh (1 med.)
Pineapple slices, canned (½ cup)
Plums, canned (½ cup), fresh (2 med.)
Tangerine (1)

Vegetables

Asparagus (½ cup)
Beets, cooked (½ cup)

Cabbage, cooked (½ cup)*
Cauliflower, cooked (½ cup)*
Celery, raw (1 cup)
Egg noodles, cooked (½ cup)
Eggplant, cooked (½ cup; remove seeds)
Mushrooms, cooked (½ cup)
Mustard greens, cooked (½ cup)
Onions, cooked (½ cup)*
Potatoes, baked, no skin (1 med.), hash browns (½ cup), mashed (½ cup)
Spinach, raw (1 cup)
String beans (½ cup)
Summer squash (½ cup)
Tomatoes, whole, remove seeds (1), canned (½ cup)
Turnips, cooked (½ cup)
Vegetable juice (1 cup)
Water chestnuts (½ cup)

Less than 1.0 gram of fiber per serving
Bread, Cereal, Rice, Pasta, and Meat Alternatives
Biscuits
Breads (1 slice): egg, French, Italian, pita (white), sourdough, white
Crackers: Melba toast (3), Saltines (4)
Dry cereal (¾ cup; check labels)
Rice cake (1)
White rice (½ cup)

Fruits
Fruit juices without pulp (½ cup)
Grapes (12)
Watermelon (1 cup)

Vegetables
Bamboo shoots, canned (½ cup)
Cucumber, peeled (½; remove seeds)
Leeks, cooked (½ cup)
Lettuce (iceberg), raw (1 cup)
Peppers, green or red, cooked (½ cup)*
Radishes (9)

*May be too gaseous for some people

Composition of Foods

The table that follows presents about 1,000 commonly eaten foods—in the forms that consumers find when shopping or dining out. The table gives the typical serving size for each food and then shows the amounts of the vital elements: calories, protein, fat (total and saturated), cholesterol, carbohydrate, fiber, and sodium. To calculate calories from fat, multiply fat grams by 9. To convert both carbohydrate and protein grams into calories, multiply by 4.

The foods are listed alphabetically within each of 14 categories. The categories are listed in the following order:

Beverages	Meat and Meat Products
Dairy Products	Mixed Dishes & Fast Foods
Eggs	Poultry & Poultry Products
Fats & Oils	Soups, Sauces, & Gravies
Fruits & Fruit Juices	Sugars & Sweets
Grain Products	Vegetables & Vegetable Products
Legumes, Nuts, & Seeds	Miscellaneous Items

Use this table to get a general idea of the nutritional value of the foods you normally eat. Check food labels for the exact amount of a particular nutrient, as brands can vary significantly. Refer to Reading Food Labels (p. 9) for further details.

Food	Amount	Calories	Protein (gm)	Total fat (gm)
BEVERAGES				
Alcoholic Beer, regular	12 oz.	146	1	0
Beer, light	12 oz.	99	1	0
Gin, rum, vodka, whiskey 80 proof	1.5 oz.	97	0	0
86 proof		105	0	0
Wine Dessert: Dry	3.5 oz.	130	Tr	0
Sweet		158	Tr	0
Table: Red		74	Tr	0
White		70	Tr	0
Carbonated Club soda	12 oz.	0	0	0
Cola	12 oz.	152	0	0
Diet cola, with aspartame	12 oz.	4	Tr	0

Saturated fat (gm)	Cholesterol (mg)	Carbohydrates (gm)	Fiber (gm)	Sodium (mg)
0	0	13	0.7	18
0	0	5	0	11
0	0	0	0	Tr
0	0	Tr	0	Tr
0	0	4	0	9
0	0	12	0	9
0	0	2	0	5
0	0	1	0	5
0	0	0	0	75
0	0	38	0	0
0	0	Tr	0	21

Food	Amount	Calories	Protein (gm)	Total fat (gm)
Carbonated *(cont'd)* Ginger ale	12 oz.	124	0	0
Grape	12 oz.	160	0	0
Lemon lime	12 oz.	147	0	0
Orange	12 oz.	179	0	0
Root beer	12 oz.	152	0	0
Chocolate-flavored beverage mix	2–3 heaping tsp.	75	1	1
Cocoa powder	3 heaping tsp.	102	3	1
Coffee, brewed	6 oz.	4	Tr	0
Coffee, instant	1 rounded tsp.	4	Tr	0
Fruit drinks, noncarbonated, ascorbic acid added Cranberry juice cocktail	8 oz.	144	0	Tr
Fruit punch	8 oz.	117	0	0

Saturated fat (gm)	Cholesterol (mg)	Carbohydrates (gm)	Fiber (gm)	Sodium (mg)
0	0	32	0	26
0	0	42	0	56
0	0	38	0	40
0	0	46	0	45
0	0	39	0	48
0.4	0	20	1.3	45
0.7	1	22	0.3	143
Tr	0	1	0	4
Tr	0	1	0	5
Tr	0	36	0.3	5
Tr	0	30	0.2	55

Food	Amount	Calories	Protein (gm)	Total fat (gm)
Fruit drinks *(cont'd)*, noncarbonated, ascorbic acid added Grape drink	8 oz.	113	0	0
Pineapple/orange juice	8 oz.	125	3	0
Lemonade, frozen concentrate	8 oz.	99	Tr	0
Lemonade, *powder* w/water	8 oz.	112	0	0
Lemonade, *powder,* low-cal.	8 oz.	5	0	0
Malted milk, powder	3 heaping tsp.	75	1	1
Milk, milk bev. *See* **Dairy Products**				
Soy milk. *See* **Legumes, Nuts, & Seeds**				
Tea, *brewed,* black	6 oz.	2	0	0
Tea, *brewed,* herb	6 oz.	2	0	0

Saturated fat (gm)	Cholesterol (mg)	Carbohydrates (gm)	Fiber (gm)	Sodium (mg)
Tr	0	29	0	15
0	0	30	0.3	8
Tr	0	26	0.2	7
Tr	0	29	0	19
0	0	1	0	7
0.4	1	18	0.2	125
Tr	0	1	0	5
Tr	0	Tr	0	2

Food	Amount	Calories	Protein (gm)	Total fat (gm)
Tea, *instant,* unsweetened	8 oz.	2	0	0
Tea, *instant,* sweetened	8 oz.	5	0	0
Water, tap	8 oz.	0	0	0

DAIRY PRODUCTS

Food	Amount	Calories	Protein (gm)	Total fat (gm)
Butter. *See* **Fats & Oils**				
Cheese *Natural* Blue	1 oz.	100	6	8
Camembert	1.3 oz.	114	8	9
Cheddar Cut pieces	1 oz.	114	7	9
Shredded	1 cup	455	28	37
Cottage 4% fat, large curd	1 cup	233	28	10
Low-fat (2%)	1 cup	203	31	4
Low-fat (1%)	1 cup	164	28	2

Saturated fat (gm)	Cholesterol (mg)	Carbohydrates (gm)	Fiber (gm)	Sodium (mg)
0	0	Tr	0	7
0	0	1	0	7
0	0	0	0	7
5.3	21	1	0	396
5.8	27	Tr	0	320
6	30	Tr	0	176
23.8	119	1	0	701
6.4	34	6	0	911
2.8	19	8	0	918
1.5	10	6	0	918

Food	Amount	Calories	Protein (gm)	Total fat (gm)
Cheese *(cont'd)*				
Natural				
Cream				
Regular	1 Tbsp.	51	1	5
Low-fat	1 Tbsp.	35	2	3
Fat-free	1 Tbsp.	15	2	Tr
Feta	1 oz.	75	4	6
Low-fat, cheddar	1 oz.	49	7	2
Mozzarella				
Whole milk	1 oz.	80	6	6
Part skim milk	1 oz.	79	8	5
Muenster	1 oz.	104	7	9
Neufchatel	1 oz.	74	3	7
Parmesan, grated	1 oz.	129	12	9
Provolone	1 oz.	100	7	8
Ricotta				
Whole milk	1 cup	428	28	32

Saturated fat (gm)	Cholesterol (mg)	Carbohydrates (gm)	Fiber (gm)	Sodium (mg)
3.2	16	Tr	0	43
1.7	8	1	0	44
0.1	1	1	0	85
4.2	25	1	0	316
1.2	6	1	0	174
3.7	22	1	0	106
3.1	15	1	0	150
5.4	27	Tr	0	178
4.2	22	1	0	113
5.4	4	Tr	0	528
4.8	20	1	0	248
20.4	124	7	0	207

Food	Amount	Calories	Protein (gm)	Total fat (gm)
Cheese *(cont'd)* *Natural* Ricotta Part skim milk	1 cup	340	28	19
Swiss	1 oz.	107	8	8
Pasteurized process American Regular	1 oz.	106	6	9
Fat-free	1 slice	31	5	Tr
Swiss	1 oz.	95	7	7
Pasteurized process cheese food, Amer.	1 oz.	93	6	7
Pasteurized process cheese food spread, Amer.	1 oz.	82	5	6
Cream, *sweet* Half and half	1 Tbsp.	20	Tr	2
Light	1 Tbsp.	29	Tr	3
Whipping, unwhipped Light	1 Tbsp.	44	Tr	5

Saturated fat (gm)	Cholesterol (mg)	Carbohydrates (gm)	Fiber (gm)	Sodium (mg)
12.1	76	13	0	307
5	26	1	0	74
5.6	27	Tr	0	406
0.1	2	3	0	321
4.5	24	1	0	388
4.4	18	2	0	337
3.8	16	2	0	381
1.1	6	1	0	6
1.8	10	1	0	6
2.9	17	Tr	0	5

Food	Amount	Calories	Protein (gm)	Total fat (gm)
Cream, *sweet (cont'd)* Whipping, unwhipped Heavy	1 Tbsp.	52	Tr	6
Whipped topping	1 Tbsp.	8	Tr	1
Cream, *sour* Regular	1 Tbsp.	26	Tr	3
Reduced-fat	1 Tbsp.	20	Tr	2
Fat-free	1 Tbsp.	12	Tr	0
Cream, *imitation* Sweet, powdered	1 Tbsp.	11	Tr	1
Whipped Topping Frozen	1 Tbsp.	13	Tr	1
Pressurized	1 Tbsp.	11	Tr	1
Sour dressing	1 Tbsp.	21	Tr	2
Frozen dessert Yogurt, soft serve Chocolate	½ cup	115	3	4
Vanilla	½ cup	114	3	4

Saturated fat (gm)	Cholesterol (mg)	Carbohydrates (gm)	Fiber (gm)	Sodium (mg)
3.5	21	Tr	0	6
0.4	2	Tr	0	4
1.6	5	1	0	6
1.1	6	1	0	6
0	1	2	0	23
0.7	0	1	0	4
0.9	0	1	0	1
0.8	0	1	0	2
1.6	1	1	0	6
2.6	4	18	1.6	71
2.5	1	17	0	63

Food	Amount	Calories	Protein (gm)	Total fat (gm)
Frozen dessert *(cont'd)*				
Ice cream				
Chocolate	½ cup	143	3	7
Vanilla	½ cup	133	2	7
Light	½ cup	92	3	3
Low-fat	½ cup	113	3	2
Soft serve, vanilla	½ cup	185	4	11
Sherbet, orange	½ cup	102	1	1
Milk, *fluid*				
Whole (3.3% fat)	1 cup	150	8	8
Reduced-fat (2%)	1 cup	121	8	5
Low-fat (1%)	1 cup	102	8	3
Nonfat (skim)	1 cup	86	8	Tr
Buttermilk	1 cup	99	8	2
Milk, *canned*				
Condensed, sweetened	1 cup	982	24	27

Saturated fat (gm)	Cholesterol (mg)	Carbohydrates (gm)	Fiber (gm)	Sodium (mg)
4.5	22	19	0.8	50
4.5	29	16	0	53
1.7	9	15	0	56
1	7	22	0.7	50
6.4	78	19	0	52
0.9	4	22	0	34
5.1	33	11	0	120
2.9	18	12	0	122
1.6	10	12	0	123
0.3	4	12	0	126
1.3	9	12	0	257
16.8	104	166	0	389

Food	Amount	Calories	Protein (gm)	Total fat (gm)
Milk, *canned* (cont'd)				
Evaporated, whole	1 cup	339	17	19
Evaporated, skim	1 cup	199	19	1
Dried				
Buttermilk	1 cup	464	41	7
Nonfat, instant	1 cup	244	24	Tr
Milk beverage				
Chocolate milk, commercial				
Whole	1 cup	208	8	8
Reduced-fat (2%)	1 cup	179	8	5
Low-fat (1%)	1 cup	158	8	3
Eggnog (commercial)	1 cup	342	10	19
Milk shake, thick				
Chocolate	10.6 oz.	356	9	8
Vanilla	11 oz.	350	12	9
Yogurt, w/low-fat milk				
Fruit-flavored	8 oz.	231	10	2

Saturated fat (gm)	Cholesterol (mg)	Carbohydrates (gm)	Fiber (gm)	Sodium (mg)
11.6	74	25	0	267
0.3	9	29	0	294
4.3	83	59	0	621
0.3	12	35	0	373
5.3	31	26	2	149
3.1	17	26	1.3	151
1.5	7	26	1.3	152
11.3	149	34	0	138
5	32	63	0.9	333
5.9	37	56	0	299
1.6	10	43	0	133

Food	Amount	Calories	Protein (gm)	Total fat (gm)
Milk beverage *(cont'd)*				
Yogurt, w/low-fat milk				
Plain	8 oz.	144	12	4
Yogurt, w/nonfat milk				
Fruit-flavored	8 oz.	213	10	Tr
Plain	8 oz.	127	13	Tr
Yogurt, w/nonfat milk, low-cal sweetener, vanilla or lemon	8 oz.	98	9	Tr

EGGS

Food	Amount	Calories	Protein (gm)	Total fat (gm)
Egg, *raw*				
Whole	1 medium	66	5	4
	1 large	75	6	5
	1 extra large	86	7	6
White	1 large	17	4	0
Yolk	1 large	59	3	5

Saturated fat (gm)	Cholesterol (mg)	Carbohydrates (gm)	Fiber (gm)	Sodium (mg)
2.3	14	16	0	159
0.3	5	43	0	132
0.3	4	17	0	174
0.3	5	17	0	134
1.4	187	1	0	55
1.6	213	1	0	63
1.8	247	1	0	73
0	0	Tr	0	55
1.6	213	Tr	0	7

Food	Amount	Calories	Protein (gm)	Total fat (gm)
Egg, *cooked,* whole Fried in margarine, w/salt	1 large	92	6	7
Hard cooked	1 large	78	6	5
Poached, w/salt	1 large	75	6	5
Scrambled, in margarine, w/salt	1 large	101	7	7
Egg substitute, liquid	¼ cup	53	8	2

FATS & OILS

Food	Amount	Calories	Protein (gm)	Total fat (gm)
Butter (4 sticks/lb) Salted	1 stick	813	1	92
	1 Tbsp.	102	Tr	12
Unsalted	1 stick	813	1	92
Lard	1 Tbsp.	115	0	13
Margarine Regular (80% fat) Hard	1 tsp.	34	Tr	4
Soft	1 tsp.	34	Tr	4

Saturated fat (gm)	Cholesterol (mg)	Carbohydrates (gm)	Fiber (gm)	Sodium (mg)
1.9	211	1	0	162
1.6	212	1	0	62
1.5	212	1	0	140
2.2	215	1	0	171
0.4	1	Tr	0	112
57.3	248	Tr	0	937
7.2	31	Tr	0	117
57.3	248	Tr	0	12
5	12	0	0	Tr
0.7	0	Tr	0	44
0.6	0	Tr	0	51

Food	Amount	Calories	Protein (gm)	Total fat (gm)
Margarine *(cont'd)* Spread (60% fat) Hard	1 tsp.	26	Tr	3
Soft	1 tsp.	26	Tr	3
Spread (40% fat)	1 tsp.	17	Tr	2
Margarine butter blend	1 Tbsp.	102	Tr	11
Oils, salad or cooking Canola	1 Tbsp.	124	0	14
Corn	1 Tbsp.	120	0	14
Olive	1 Tbsp.	119	0	14
Peanut	1 Tbsp.	119	0	14
Safflower	1 Tbsp.	120	0	14
Sesame	1 Tbsp.	120	0	14
Soybean, hydrogenated	1 Tbsp.	120	0	14
Soybean/cottonseed blend	1 Tbsp.	120	0	14

Saturated fat (gm)	Cholesterol (mg)	Carbohydrates (gm)	Fiber (gm)	Sodium (mg)
0.7	0	0	0	48
0.6	0	0	0	48
0.4	0	Tr	0	46
4	12	Tr	0	127
1	0	0	0	0
1.7	0	0	0	0
1.8	0	0	0	Tr
2.3	0	0	0	Tr
0.8	0	0	0	0
1.9	0	0	0	0
2	0	0	0	0
2/4	0	0	0	0

Food	Amount	Calories	Protein (gm)	Total fat (gm)
Oils, salad or cooking *(cont'd)*				
Sunflower	1 Tbsp.	120	0	14
Salad dressings, *commercial*				
Blue cheese				
Regular	1 Tbsp.	77	1	8
Low Calorie	1 Tbsp.	15	1	1
Caesar				
Regular	1 Tbsp.	78	Tr	8
Low-Calorie	1 Tbsp.	17	Tr	1
French				
Regular	1 Tbsp.	67	Tr	6
Low-Calorie	1 Tbsp.	22	Tr	4
Italian				
Regular	1 Tbsp.	69	Tr	7
Low-Calorie	1 Tbsp.	16	Tr	1
Mayonnaise				
Regular	1 Tbsp.	99	Tr	11
Light, cholesterol-free	1 Tbsp.	49	Tr	5

Saturated fat (gm)	Cholesterol (mg)	Carbohydrates (gm)	Fiber (gm)	Sodium (mg)
1.4	0	0	0	0
1.5	3	1	0	167
0.4	Tr	Tr	0	184
1.3	Tr	Tr	Tr	158
0.1	Tr	3	Tr	162
1.5	0	3	0	214
0.1	0	4	0	128
1	0	1	0	116
0.2	1	1	Tr	118
1.6	8	Tr	0	78
0.7	0	1	0	107

Food	Amount	Calories	Protein (gm)	Total fat (gm)
Salad dressings, commercial *(cont'd)* Mayonnaise Fat-free	1 Tbsp.	12	0	Tr
Russian Regular	1 Tbsp.	76	Tr	8
Low-Calorie	1 Tbsp.	23	Tr	1
Thousand Island Regular	1 Tbsp.	59	Tr	6
Low-Calorie	1 Tbsp.	24	Tr	2
Salad dressings, home recipe Cooked, w/margarine	1 Tbsp.	25	1	2
French	1 Tbsp.	88	Tr	10
Vinegar & Oil	1 Tbsp.	70	0	8
Shortening	1 Tbsp.	113	0	13

FISH & SHELLFISH

Food	Amount	Calories	Protein (gm)	Total fat (gm)
Catfish, fried	3 oz.	195	15	11

Saturated fat (gm)	Cholesterol (mg)	Carbohydrates (gm)	Fiber (gm)	Sodium (mg)
0.1	0	2	0.6	190
1.1	3	2	0	133
0.1	1	4	Tr	141
0.9	4	2	0	109
0.2	2	2	0.2	153
0.5	9	2	0	117
1.8	0	Tr	0	92
1.4	0	Tr	0	Tr
3.2	0	0	0	0
2.8	69	7	0.6	238

Food	Amount	Calories	Protein (gm)	Total fat (gm)
Clam, raw	1 medium	11	2	Tr
Clam, fried	¾ cup	451	13	26
Cod, baked/broiled	3 oz.	89	20	1
Crab Alaska king, steamed	3 oz.	82	16	1
Imitation; surimi	3 oz.	87	10	1
Blue, steamed	3 oz.	87	17	2
Crab cake	1 cake	93	12	5
Flounder or sole, baked or broiled	3 oz.	99	21	1
Haddock, baked or broiled	3 oz.	95	21	1
Halibut, baked or broiled	3 oz.	119	23	2
Herring, pickled	3 oz.	223	12	15
Lobster, steamed	3 oz.	83	17	1
Oyster, *raw*	6 medium	169	17	6

Saturated fat (gm)	Cholesterol (mg)	Carbohydrates (gm)	Fiber (gm)	Sodium (mg)
Tr	5	Tr	0	8
6.6	87	39	0.3	834
0.1	40	0	0	77
0.1	45	0	0	911
0.2	17	9	0	715
0.2	85	0	0	237
0.9	90	Tr	0	198
0.3	58	0	0	89
0.1	63	0	0	74
0.4	35	0	0	59
2	11	8	0	740
0.1	61	1	0	323
0.6	45	3	0	177

Food	Amount	Calories	Protein (gm)	Total fat (gm)
Oyster, *breaded,* fried	3 oz.	167	7	11
Pollock, baked or broiled	3 oz.	96	20	1
Salmon Baked or broiled	3 oz.	184	23	9
Canned	3 oz.	118	17	5
Smoked	3 oz.	99	16	4
Sardine, Atlantic	3 oz.	177	21	10
Scallop, steamed	3 oz.	95	20	1
Shrimp, breaded/fried	6 large	109	10	6
Swordfish, baked or broiled	3 oz.	132	22	4
Trout, baked or broiled	3 oz.	144	21	6
Tuna Baked or broiled	3 oz.	118	25	1
Canned, oil pack	3 oz.	168	25	7

Saturated fat (gm)	Cholesterol (mg)	Carbohydrates (gm)	Fiber (gm)	Sodium (mg)
2.7	69	10	0.2	354
0.2	82	0	0	99
1.6	74	0	0	56
1.3	47	0	0	471
0.8	20	0	0	666
1.3	121	0	0	429
0.1	45	3	0	225
0.9	80	5	0.2	155
1.2	43	0	0	98
1.8	58	0	0	36
0.3	49	0	0	40
1.3	15	0	0	301

Food	Amount	Calories	Protein (gm)	Total fat (gm)
Tuna *(cont'd)* Canned, water pack	3 oz.	99	22	1
Tuna salad, mayo-type dressing	1 cup	383	33	19

FRUITS & FRUIT JUICES

Food	Amount	Calories	Protein (gm)	Total fat (gm)
Apples Raw	1 apple	81	Tr	Tr
Peeled, sliced	1 cup	63	Tr	Tr
Apple juice	1 cup	117	Tr	Tr
Apple pie filling	2.6 oz.	75	Tr	Tr
Applesauce Sweetened	1 cup	194	Tr	Tr
Unsweetened	1 cup	105	Tr	Tr
Apricots Raw, pitted	1 apricot	17	Tr	Tr
Canned, heavy syrup	1 cup	214	1	Tr
Avocados California	1 oz.	50	1	5

Saturated fat (gm)	Cholesterol (mg)	Carbohydrates (gm)	Fiber (gm)	Sodium (mg)
0.2	26	0	0	287
3.2	27	19	0	824
0.1	0	21	0.7	0
0.1	0	16	2.1	0
Tr	0	29	0.2	7
Tr	0	19	0.7	33
0.1	0	51	3.1	8
Tr	0	28	0.9	5
Tr	0	4	0.8	Tr
Tr	0	55	4.1	10
0.7	0	2	1.4	3

Food	Amount	Calories	Protein (gm)	Total fat (gm)
Avocados (cont'd) Florida	1 oz.	32	Tr	3
Bananas	1 med.	109	1	1
Blackberries	1 cup	75	1	1
Blueberries	1 cup	81	1	1
Cantaloupe. *See* **Melons**				
Cherries Sour, red, canned	1 cup	88	2	Tr
Sweet, raw pitted	10 cherries	49	1	1
Cherry pie filling, canned	4.2 oz.	85	Tr	Tr
Cranberries, dried	¼ cup	92	Tr	Tr
Cranberry sauce, canned	1 slice	86	Tr	Tr
Dates, pitted, whole	5 dates	116	1	Tr
Figs, dried	2 figs	97	1	Tr

Saturated fat (gm)	Cholesterol (mg)	Carbohydrates (gm)	Fiber (gm)	Sodium (mg)
0.5	0	3	1.5	1
0.2	0	28	2.8	1
Tr	0	18	7.6	0
Tr	0	20	3.9	9
0.1	0	22	2.7	17
0.1	0	11	1.6	0
Tr	0	21	0.4	13
Tr	0	24	2.5	1
Tr	0	22	0.6	17
0.1	0	31	3.2	1
0.1	0	25	4.6	4

Food	Amount	Calories	Protein (gm)	Total fat (gm)
Fruit cocktail, canned, heavy syrup	1 cup	181	1	Tr
Grapefruit Pink or red	½ grapefruit	37	1	Tr
White	½ grapefruit	39	1	Tr
Canned, light syrup	1 cup	152	1	Tr
Grapefruit juice Unsweetened	1 cup	94	1	Tr
Sweetened	1 cup	115	1	Tr
Grapes, seedless	10 grapes	36	Tr	Tr
Grape juice Canned or bottled	1 cup	154	1	Tr
Frozen concentrate, w/3 parts water	1 cup	128	Tr	Tr
Kiwi, w/o skin	1 med.	46	1	Tr
Lemons	1 lemon	17	1	Tr
Lemon juice, unsweetened	1 Tbsp.	3	Tr	Tr

Saturated fat (gm)	Cholesterol (mg)	Carbohydrates (gm)	Fiber (gm)	Sodium (mg)
Tr	0	47	2.5	15
Tr	0	9	1.4	0
Tr	0	10	1.3	0
Tr	0	39	1	5
Tr	0	22	0.2	2
Tr	0	28	0.3	5
0.1	0	9	0.5	1
0.1	0	38	0.3	8
0.1	0	32	0.3	5
Tr	0	11	2.6	4
Tr	0	5	1.6	1
Tr	0	1	0.1	3

Food	Amount	Calories	Protein (gm)	Total fat (gm)
Lime juice, unsweetened	1 Tbsp.	3	Tr	Tr
Mangos	1 mango	135	1	1
Melons Cantaloupe	⅛ melon	24	1	Tr
Honeydew	⅛ melon	56	1	Tr
Nectarines	1 nectarine	67	1	1
Oranges	1 orange	62	1	Tr
Orange juice Raw	1 cup	112	2	Tr
Chilled	1 cup	110	2	1
Frozen concentrate, w/3 parts water	1 cup	112	2	Tr
Papayas	1 papaya	119	2	Tr
Peaches Raw	1 peach	42	1	Tr
Canned, heavy syrup	1 cup	194	1	Tr

Saturated fat (gm)	Cholesterol (mg)	Carbohydrates (gm)	Fiber (gm)	Sodium (mg)
Tr	0	1	0.1	2
0.1	0	35	3.7	4
Tr	0	6	0.6	6
Tr	0	15	1	16
0.1	0	16	2.2	0
Tr	0	15	3.1	0
0.1	0	26	0.5	2
0.1	0	25	0.5	2
Tr	0	27	0.5	2
0.1	0	30	5.5	9
Tr	0	11	2	0
Tr	0	52	3.4	16

Food	Amount	Calories	Protein (gm)	Total fat (gm)
Pears Raw, cored	1 pear	98	1	1
Canned, heavy syrup	1 cup	197	1	Tr
Pineapple Raw, diced	1 cup	76	1	1
Canned, heavy syrup	1 cup	198	1	Tr
Pineapple juice, canned, unsweetened	1 cup	140	1	Tr
Plantain, raw, peeled	1 med.	218	2	1
Plums Raw	1 plum	36	1	Tr
Canned, heavy syrup	1 cup	230	1	Tr
Prunes, dried, pitted Uncooked	5 prunes	100	1	Tr
Stewed	1 cup	265	3	1
Prune juice	1 cup	182	2	Tr
Raisins, seedless	1 cup	435	5	1

Saturated fat (gm)	Cholesterol (mg)	Carbohydrates (gm)	Fiber (gm)	Sodium (mg)
Tr	0	25	4	0
Tr	0	51	4.3	13
Tr	0	19	1.9	2
Tr	0	51	2	3
Tr	0	34	0.5	3
0.3	0	57	4.1	7
Tr	0	9	1	0
Tr	0	60	2.6	49
Tr	0	26	3	2
Tr	0	70	16.4	5
Tr	0	45	2.6	10
0.2	0	115	5.8	17

Food	Amount	Calories	Protein (gm)	Total fat (gm)
Raspberries Raw	1 cup	60	1	1
Frozen, sweetened	1 cup	258	2	Tr
Rhubarb, frozen, w/sugar	1 cup	278	1	Tr
Strawberries Raw, large	1 berry	5	Tr	Tr
Frozen, sweetened, sliced	1 cup	245	1	Tr
Tangerines	1 tangerine	37	1	Tr
Watermelon	1 cup	49	1	1

GRAIN PRODUCTS

Food	Amount	Calories	Protein (gm)	Total fat (gm)
Bagels, plain, 3½"	1 bagel	195	7	1
Banana bread	1 slice	196	3	6
Barley, pearled	1 cup	193	4	1
Biscuits, plain or buttermilk w/2% milk	1 biscuit	212	4	10

Saturated fat (gm)	Cholesterol (mg)	Carbohydrates (gm)	Fiber (gm)	Sodium (mg)
Tr	0	14	8.4	0
Tr	0	65	11	3
Tr	0	75	4.8	2
Tr	0	1	0.4	Tr
Tr	0	66	4.8	8
Tr	0	9	1.9	1
0.1	0	11	0.8	3
0.2	0	38	1.6	379
1.3	26	33	0.7	181
0.1	0	155	31.2	18
2.6	2	27	0.9	348

Food	Amount	Calories	Protein (gm)	Total fat (gm)
Biscuits, plain or buttermilk *(cont'd)* Refrig. dough	1 biscuit	93	2	4
Breads, enriched Cracked wheat	1 slice	65	2	1
French, Vienna, sourdough	½ slice	69	2	1
Italian	1 slice	54	2	1
Mixed-grain	1 slice	65	3	1
Oatmeal	1 slice	73	2	1
Pita	4" pita	77	3	Tr
Pumpernickel	1 slice	80	3	1
Raisin	1 slice	71	2	1
Rye	1 slice	83	3	1
Rye, reduced-cal.	1 slice	47	2	1
Wheat	1 slice	65	2	1
Wheat, reduced-cal.	1 slice	46	2	1

Saturated fat (gm)	Cholesterol (mg)	Carbohydrates (gm)	Fiber (gm)	Sodium (mg)
1	0	13	0.4	325
0.2	0	12	1.4	135
0.2	0	13	0.8	152
0.2	0	10	0.5	117
0.2	0	12	1.7	127
0.2	0	13	1.1	162
Tr	0	16	0.6	150
0.1	0	15	2.1	215
0.3	0	14	1.1	101
0.2	0	15	0.9	211
0.1	0	9	2.8	93
0.2	0	12	1.1	133
0.1	0	10	2.8	118

Food	Amount	Calories	Protein (gm)	Total fat (gm)
Breads, enriched *(cont'd)*				
White	1 slice	67	2	1
White, reduced-cal.	1 slice	48	2	1
Bread, whole wheat	1 slice	69	3	1
Bread crumbs				
Plain, enriched	1 cup	427	14	6
Seasoned	1 cup	440	17	3
Breakfast bar, fat-free, fruit filling	1 bar	121	2	Tr
Breakfast cereals				
Hot type, cooked				
Corn grits, white, reg., or quick	1 cup	145	3	Tr
Grits, instant	1 packet	89	2	Tr
Cream of Wheat, quick	1 cup	129	4	Tr
Oatmeal				
Regular, quick, or instant, plain	1 cup	145	6	2
Instant, fortified	1 packet	104	4	2

Saturated fat (gm)	Cholesterol (mg)	Carbohydrates (gm)	Fiber (gm)	Sodium (mg)
0.1	Tr	12	0.6	135
0.1	0	10	2.2	104
0.3	0	13	1.9	148
1.3	0	78	0.6	931
0.9	1	84	5	3,180
Tr	Tr	28	0.8	203
0.1	0	31	0.5	0
Tr	0	21	1.2	289
0.1	0	27	1.2	139
0.4	0	25	4	2
0.3	0	18	3	285

Food	Amount	Calories	Protein (gm)	Total fat (gm)
Breakfast cereals *(cont'd)*				
Oatmeal				
Quaker instant				
Apples, cinnamon	1 packet	125	3	1
Maple, brown sugar	1 packet	153	4	2
Wheatena	1 cup	136	5	1
Ready-to-eat				
All Bran	½ cup	79	4	1
Applejacks	1 cup	116	1	Tr
Cap'n Crunch	¾ cup	107	1	1
Cheerios	1 cup	110	3	2
Chex				
Corn	1 cup	113	2	Tr
Honey-nut	¾ cup	117	2	1
Wheat	1 cup	104	3	1
Cocoa Puffs	1 cup	119	1	1

Saturated fat (gm)	Cholesterol (mg)	Carbohydrates (gm)	Fiber (gm)	Sodium (mg)
0.3	0	26	2.5	121
0.4	0	31	2.6	234
0.2	0	29	6.6	5
0.2	0	23	9.7	61
0.1	0	27	0.6	134
0.4	0	23	0.0	208
0.4	0	23	2.6	284
0.1	0	26	0.5	289
0.1	0	26	0.4	224
0.1	0	24	3.3	269
0.2	0	27	0.2	181

Food	Amount	Calories	Protein (gm)	Total fat (gm)
Breakfast cereals *(cont'd)*				
Corn Flakes				
General Mills, Total	1⅓ cup	112	2	Tr
Kellogg's	1 cup	102	2	Tr
Corn Pops	1 cup	118	1	Tr
Crispix	1 cup	108	2	Tr
Froot Loops	1 cup	117	1	1
Frosted Flakes	¾ cup	119	1	Tr
Frosted Mini Wheats, reg.	1 cup	173	5	1
Honey Nut Cheerios	1 cup	115	3	1
Kix	1⅓ cup	114	2	1
Life	¾ cup	121	3	1
Nature Valley Granola	¾ cup	248	6	10
Product 19	1 cup	110	3	Tr

Saturated fat (gm)	Cholesterol (mg)	Carbohydrates (gm)	Fiber (gm)	Sodium (mg)
0.2	0	26	0.8	203
0.1	0	24	0.8	298
0.1	0	28	0.4	123
0.1	0	25	0.6	240
0.4	0	26	0.6	141
0.1	0	28	0.6	200
0.2	0	42	5.5	2
0.2	0	24	1.6	259
0.2	0	26	0.8	263
0.2	0	25	2	174
1.3	0	36	3.5	69
Tr	0	25	1	216

Food	Amount	Calories	Protein (gm)	Total fat (gm)
Breakfast cereals *(cont'd)*				
Puffed Rice	1 cup	56	1	Tr
Puffed Wheat	1 cup	44	2	Tr
Raisin Bran General Mills	1 cup	178	4	1
Kellogg's	1 cup	186	6	1
Rice Krispies	1¼ cup	124	2	Tr
Shredded Wheat	2 biscuits	156	5	1
Special K	1 cup	115	6	Tr
Total	¾ cup	105	3	1
Trix	1 cup	122	1	2
Wheaties	1 cup	110	3	1
Brownies Regular, large	1 brownie	227	3	9
Fat-free	1 brownie	89	1	Tr
Buckwheat flour	1 cup	402	15	4

Saturated fat (gm)	Cholesterol (mg)	Carbohydrates (gm)	Fiber (gm)	Sodium (mg)
Tr	0	13	0.2	Tr
Tr	0	10	0.5	Tr
0.2	0	43	5	240
0	0	47	8.2	354
0.1	0	29	0.4	354
0.1	0	38	5.3	3
0	0	22	1	250
0.2	Tr	39	3.3	185
0.4	0	24	2.6	199
0.2	0	24	2.1	222
2.4	10	36	1.2	175
0.2	0	22	1.2	90
0.8	0	16	0.8	21

Food	Amount	Calories	Protein (gm)	Total fat (gm)
Bulgur, cooked	1 cup	151	6	Tr
Cakes, *from dry mix* Angel food	1 piece	129	3	Tr
Yellow, light	1 piece	181	3	2
Cakes, *from recipe* Chocolate	1 piece	340	5	14
Gingerbread	1 piece	263	3	12
Pineapple upside down	1 piece	367	4	14
Shortcake	1 shortcake	225	4	9
Sponge, white	1 piece	187	5	3
Cakes, *commercial* Angel food	1 piece	72	2	Tr
Boston cream	1 piece	232	2	8
Chocolate, w/choc. frosting	1 piece	235	3	10
Coffee cake	1 piece	263	4	15

Saturated fat (gm)	Cholesterol (mg)	Carbohydrates (gm)	Fiber (gm)	Sodium (mg)
0.1	0	34	8.2	9
Tr	0	29	0.1	255
1.1	0	37	0.6	279
5.2	55	51	1.5	299
3.1	24	36	0.7	242
3.4	25	58	0.9	367
2.5	2	32	0.8	329
0.8	107	36	0.4	144
Tr	0	16	0.4	210
2.2	34	39	1.3	132
3.1	27	35	1.8	214
3.7	20	29	1.3	221

Food	Amount	Calories	Protein (gm)	Total fat (gm)
Cakes, *commercial* (cont'd)				
Fruitcake	1 piece	139	1	4
Pound				
Butter	1 piece	109	2	6
Fat-free	1 slice	79	2	Tr
Snack cakes				
Chocolate, crème-filled, w/frosting	1 cupcake	188	2	7
Chocolate, w/ frosting, low-fat	1 cupcake	131	2	2
Sponge, crème-filled	1 cake	155	1	5
Yellow, w/chocolate frosting	1 piece	243	2	11
Cheesecake	1 piece	257	4	18
Cheese flavor puffs/twists	1 oz.	157	2	10
Cookies				
Butter	1 cookie	23	Tr	1

Saturated fat (gm)	Cholesterol (mg)	Carbohydrates (gm)	Fiber (gm)	Sodium (mg)
0.5	2	26	1.6	116
3.2	62	14	0.1	111
0.1	0	17	0.3	95
1.4	9	30	0.4	213
0.5	0	29	1.8	178
1.1	7	27	0.2	155
3	35	35	1.2	216
7.9	44	20	0.3	166
1.9	1	15	0.3	298
0.6	6	3	Tr	18

Food	Amount	Calories	Protein (gm)	Total fat (gm)
Cookies *(cont'd)* Chocolate chip, med. Regular	1 cookie	48	1	2
Reduced-fat	1 cookie	45	1	2
Refrig. dough	1 cookie	128	1	6
Recipe	1 cookie	78	1	5
Devil's food, fat-free	1 cookie	49	1	Tr
Fig bar	1 cookie	56	1	1
Molasses, med.	1 cookie	65	1	2
Oatmeal Regular, large	1 cookie	113	2	5
Soft type	1 cookie	61	1	2
Fat-free	1 cookie	36	1	Tr
From recipe	1 cookie	65	1	2
Peanut Butter Commercial	1 cookie	72	1	4
From recipe	1 cookie	95	2	5

Saturated fat (gm)	Cholesterol (mg)	Carbohydrates (gm)	Fiber (gm)	Sodium (mg)
0.7	0	7	0.3	32
0.4	0	7	0.4	38
2	7	18	0.4	60
1.3	5	9	0.4	58
0.1	0	12	0.3	28
0.2	0	11	0.7	56
0.5	0	11	0.1	69
1.1	0	17	0.7	96
0.5	1	10	0.4	52
Tr	0	9	0.8	33
0.5	5	10	0.5	81
0.7	Tr	9	0.3	62
0.9	6	12	0.4	104

Food	Amount	Calories	Protein (gm)	Total fat (gm)
Cookies *(cont'd)* Sandwich-type, crème filling Chocolate	1 cookie	47	Tr	2
Vanilla	1 cookie	48	Tr	2
Shortbread, plain	1 cookie	40	Tr	2
Sugar Commercial	1 cookie	72	1	3
From recipe	1 cookie	66	1	3
Vanilla wafer	1 cookie	18	Tr	1
Cornbread From mix	1 piece	188	4	6
From recipe	1 piece	173	4	5
Corn chips	1 oz.	153	2	9
Cornmeal, yellow, whole grain	1 cup	442	10	4
Cornstarch	1 Tbsp.	30	Tr	Tr
Couscous, cooked	1 cup	176	6	Tr

Saturated fat (gm)	Cholesterol (mg)	Carbohydrates (gm)	Fiber (gm)	Sodium (mg)
0.4	0	7	0.3	60
0.3	0	7	0.2	35
0.5	2	5	0.1	36
0.8	8	10	0.1	54
0.7	4	8	0.2	69
0.2	2	3	0.1	12
1.6	37	29	1.4	467
1	26	28	1.9	428
1.3	0	16	1.4	179
0.6	0	94	8.9	43
Tr	0	7	0.1	1
Tr	0	36	2.2	8

Food	Amount	Calories	Protein (gm)	Total fat (gm)
Crackers Cheese, 1″ sq.	10 crackers	50	1	3
Graham, plain	2 sq.	59	1	1
Melba toast	4 pieces	78	2	1
Rye wafer	1 wafer	37	1	Tr
Saltine Square	4 crackers	52	1	1
Oyster type	1 cup	195	4	5
Sandwich type Wheat w/cheese	1 sand- wich	33	1	1
Cheese w/peanut butter	1 sand- wich	34	1	2
Wheat, thin square	4 crackers	38	1	2
Whole wheat	4 crackers	71	1	3
Croissant, butter	1 croissant	231	5	12
Croutons, seasoned	1 cup	186	4	7

Saturated fat (gm)	Cholesterol (mg)	Carbohydrates (gm)	Fiber (gm)	Sodium (mg)
0.9	1	6	0.2	100
0.2	0	11	0.4	85
0.1	0	15	1.3	166
Tr	0	9	2.5	87
0.4	0	9	0.4	156
1.3	0	32	1.4	586
0.4	Tr	4	0.1	98
0.4	Tr	4	0.2	69
0.4	0	5	0.4	64
0.5	0	11	1.7	105
6.6	38	26	1.5	424
2.1	3	25	2	495

Food	Amount	Calories	Protein (gm)	Total fat (gm)
Danish pastry, enriched Cheese-filled	1 Danish	266	6	16
Fruit-filled	1 Danish	263	4	13
Doughnuts Cake-type	1 med.	198	2	11
Glazed	1 med.	242	4	14
Éclair, from recipe	1 éclair	262	6	16
English muffin, plain	1 muffin	134	4	1
French toast	1 slice	149	5	7
Granola bar, plain	1 bar	134	3	6
Macaroni, cooked	1 cup	197	7	1
Matzo, plain	1 matzo	112	3	Tr
Muffins Blueberry, commercial	1 muffin	158	3	4
Blueberry, from recipe	1 muffin	162	4	6

Saturated fat (gm)	Cholesterol (mg)	Carbohydrates (gm)	Fiber (gm)	Sodium (mg)
4.8	11	26	0.7	320
3.5	81	34	1.3	251
1.7	17	23	0.7	257
3.5	4	27	0.7	205
4.1	127	24	0.6	337
0.1	0	26	1.5	264
1.8	75	16	0.7	311
0.7	0	18	1.5	83
0.1	0	40	1.8	1
0.1	0	24	0.9	1
0.8	17	27	1.5	255
1.2	21	23	1.1	251

Food	Amount	Calories	Protein (gm)	Total fat (gm)
Muffins *(cont'd)* Bran, w/raisins	1 muffin	106	2	3
Corn	1 muffin	174	3	5
Oat bran	1 muffin	154	4	4
Noodles, enriched Regular	1 cup	213	8	2
Spinach	1 cup	211	8	2
NutriGrain cereal bar, fruit-filled	1 bar	136	2	3
Oat bran, cooked	1 cup	88	7	2
Pancakes, plain, 4″ diam. Frozen	1 pancake	82	2	1
From mix	1 pancake	74	2	1
Pie crust, baked, standard From recipe	1 pie shell	949	12	62
From frozen	1 pie shell	648	6	41

Saturated fat (gm)	Cholesterol (mg)	Carbohydrates (gm)	Fiber (gm)	Sodium (mg)
0.5	3	19	2.8	179
0.8	15	29	1.9	297
0.6	0	28	2.6	224
0.5	53	40	1.8	11
0.6	53	39	3.7	19
0.6	0	27	0.8	110
0.4	0	25	5.7	2
0.3	3	16	0.6	183
0.2	5	14	0.5	239
15.5	0	86	3	976
13.3	0	62	1.3	815

Food	Amount	Calories	Protein (gm)	Total fat (gm)
Pies Commercial (⅙ of 8″ diam.) Apple	1 piece	277	2	13
Blueberry	1 piece	271	2	12
Cherry	1 piece	304	2	13
Choc. crème	1 piece	344	3	22
Lemon meringue	1 piece	303	2	10
Pecan	1 piece	452	5	21
Pumpkin	1 piece	229	4	10
Popcorn Air-popped, unsalted	1 cup	31	1	Tr
Oil-popped, salted	1 cup	55	1	3
Cheese-flavored	1 cup	58	1	4
Pretzels, w/enriched flour Stick, 2¼″	10 pretzels	11	Tr	Tr
Twisted	10 pretzels	229	5	2

Saturated fat (gm)	Cholesterol (mg)	Carbohydrates (gm)	Fiber (gm)	Sodium (mg)
4.4	0	40	1.9	311
2	0	41	1.2	380
3	0	47	0.9	288
5.6	6	38	2.3	154
2	51	53	1.4	165
4	36	65	4	479
1.9	22	30	2.9	307
Tr	0	6	1.2	Tr
0.5	0	6	1.1	97
0.7	1	6	1.1	98
Tr	0	2	0.1	51
0.5	0	48	1.9	1,029

Food	Amount	Calories	Protein (gm)	Total fat (gm)
Rice Brown, cooked	1 cup	216	5	2
White, cooked	1 cup	205	4	Tr
Instant, prepared	1 cup	162	3	Tr
Wild, cooked		166	7	1
Rice cake, brown rice	1 cake	35	1	Tr
Rolls Dinner	1 roll	84	2	2
Hamburger/hotdog	1 roll	123	4	2
Hard, Kaiser	1 roll	167	6	2
Spaghetti, cooked	1 cup	187	7	1
Taco shell, baked	1 med.	62	1	3
Tapioca, dry	1 cup	544	Tr	Tr
Tortilla chips Plain	1 oz.	142	2	7
Nacho	1 oz.	141	2	7

Saturated fat (gm)	Cholesterol (mg)	Carbohydrates (gm)	Fiber (gm)	Sodium (mg)
0.4	0	45	3.5	10
0.1	0	45	0.6	2
0.1	0	35	1	5
0.1	0	35	3	5
0.1	0	7	0.4	29
0.5	Tr	14	0.8	146
0.5	0	22	1.2	241
0.3	0	30	1.3	310
0.1	0	40	2.4	1
0.4	0	8	1	49
Tr	0	135	1.4	2
1.4	0	18	1.8	150
1.4	1	18	1.5	201

Food	Amount	Calories	Protein (gm)	Total fat (gm)
Tortilla chips *(cont'd)*				
Nacho, reduced-fat	1 oz.	126	2	4
Tortillas, ready-to-cook, 6″ diam.				
Corn	1 tortilla	58	1	1
Flour	1 tortilla	104	3	2
Waffles, plain				
From recipe, 7″ diam.	1 waffle	218	6	11
Frozen, toasted, 4″ diam.	1 waffle	87	2	3
Low-fat, 4″ diam.	1 waffle	83	2	1
Wheat flour				
All-purpose, enriched, sifted	1 cup	419	12	1
Bread, enriched	1 cup	495	16	2
Cake or pastry	1 cup	496	11	1
Self-rising, enriched	1 cup	443	12	1
Wheat germ, toasted, plain	1 Tbsp.	27	2	1

Saturated fat (gm)	Cholesterol (mg)	Carbohydrates (gm)	Fiber (gm)	Sodium (mg)
0.8	1	20	1.4	284
0.1	0	12	1.4	42
0.6	0	18	1.1	153
2.1	52	25	0.7	383
0.5	8	13	0.8	260
0.3	9	15	0.4	155
0.2	0	88	3.1	2
0.3	0	99	3.3	3
0.2	0	107	2.3	3
0.2	0	93	3.4	1,588
0.1	0	3	0.9	Tr

Food	Amount	Calories	Protein (gm)	Total fat (gm)
LEGUMES, NUTS, & SEEDS				
Almonds, shelled, whole	1 oz.	164	6	14
Beans, dry *Cooked* Black	1 cup	227	15	1
Great Northern	1 cup	205	15	1
Kidney, Red	1 cup	225	15	1
Lima, large	1 cup	216	15	1
Pea (navy)	1 cup	258	16	1
Pinto	1 cup	234	14	1
Canned Baked beans Plain or veg.	1 cup	236	12	1
w/hot dogs	1 cup	368	17	17
w/pork in tomato sauce	1 cup	248	13	3
Kidney, red	1 cup	218	13	1

Saturated fat (gm)	Cholesterol (mg)	Carbohydrates (gm)	Fiber (gm)	Sodium (mg)
1.1	0	6	3.3	Tr
0.2	0	41	15	2
0.2	0	37	12.4	4
0.1	0	40	13.1	4
0.2	0	39	13.2	4
0.3	0	48	11.6	2
0.2	0	44	14.7	3
0.3	0	52	12.7	1,008
6.1	16	40	17.9	1,114
1	18	49	12.1	1,113
0.1	0	40	16.4	873

Food	Amount	Calories	Protein (gm)	Total fat (gm)
Beans, dry *(cont'd)*				
Canned				
Lima, large	1 cup	190	12	Tr
White	1 cup	307	19	1
Black-eyed peas, cooked	1 cup	200	13	1
Brazil nuts, shelled	1 oz.	186	4	19
Cashews, salted				
Dry-roasted	1 oz.	163	4	13
Oil-roasted	1 oz.	163	5	14
Coconut, raw, shredded	1 cup	283	3	27
Hummus	1 Tbsp.	23	1	1
Lentils, cooked	1 cup	230	18	1
Macadamia nuts, dry-roasted, salted	1 oz.	203	2	22
Mixed nuts, salted				
Dry-roasted	1 oz.	168	5	15
Oil-roasted	1 oz.	175	5	16

Saturated fat (gm)	Cholesterol (mg)	Carbohydrates (gm)	Fiber (gm)	Sodium (mg)
0.1	0	36	11.6	810
0.2	0	57	12.6	13
0.2	0	36	11.2	7
4.6	0	4	1.5	1
2.6	0	9	0.9	181
2.7	0	8	1.1	177
23.8	0	12	7.2	16
0.2	0	2	0.8	53
0.1	0	40	15.6	4
3.4	0	4	2.3	75
2	0	7	2.6	190
2.5	0	6	2.6	185

Food	Amount	Calories	Protein (gm)	Total fat (gm)
Peanuts Dry-roasted	1 oz.	166	7	14
Dry-roasted, unsalted	1 oz.	166	7	14
Oil-roasted, salted	1 oz.	165	7	14
Peanut butter Regular, smooth	1 Tbsp.	95	4	8
Regular, chunk	1 Tbsp.	94	4	8
Reduced-fat, smooth	1 Tbsp.	94	5	6
Peas, split, cooked	1 cup	231	16	1
Pecans, halves	1 oz.	196	3	20
Pistachio nuts, shelled, salted	1 oz.	161	6	13
Refried beans, canned	1 cup	237	14	3
Soybeans, cooked	1 cup	298	29	15
Soy products Miso	1 cup	567	32	17

Saturated fat (gm)	Cholesterol (mg)	Carbohydrates (gm)	Fiber (gm)	Sodium (mg)
2	0	6	2.3	230
2	0	6	2.3	2
1.9	0	5	2.6	123
1.7	0	3	0.9	75
1.5	0	3	1.1	78
1.3	0	6	0.9	97
0.1	0	41	16.3	4
1.8	0	4	2.7	0
1.6	0	8	2.9	121
1.2	20	39	13.4	753
2.2	0	17	10.3	2
2.4	0	77	14.9	10,029

Food	Amount	Calories	Protein (gm)	Total fat (gm)
Soy products *(cont'd)* Soy milk	1 cup	81	7	5
Tofu, firm	¼ block	62	7	4
Sunflower seed kernels, dry-roasted, salted	1 oz.	165	5	14
Walnuts, English	1 oz.	185	4	18

MEAT & MEAT PRODUCTS

Food	Amount	Calories	Protein (gm)	Total fat (gm)
Beef, *cooked* Braised, simmered, or pot roasted Relatively fat cut Lean and fat	3 oz.	293	23	22
Relatively lean cut Lean and fat	3 oz.	234	24	14
Ground beef, broiled 83% lean	3 oz.	218	22	14
73% lean	3 oz.	246	20	18
Liver, fried	3 oz.	184	23	7

Saturated fat (gm)	Cholesterol (mg)	Carbohydrates (gm)	Fiber (gm)	Sodium (mg)
0.5	0	4	3.2	29
0.5	0	2	0.3	6
1.5	0	7	2.6	221
1.7	0	4	1.9	1
8.7	88	0	0	54
5.4	82	0	0	43
5.5	71	0	0	60
6.9	77	0	0	71
2.3	410	7	0	90

Food	Amount	Calories	Protein (gm)	Total fat (gm)
Beef, *cooked (cont'd)* Roast Relatively fat cut Lean & fat	3 oz.	304	19	25
Relatively lean cut Lean & fat	3 oz.	195	23	11
Steak, sirloin, lean & fat	3 oz.	219	24	13
Beef, *canned,* corned	3 oz.	213	23	13
Beef, *chipped*	1 oz.	47	8	1
Lamb, cooked Chops, arm, braised Lean and fat	3 oz.	294	26	20
Chops, loin, broiled Lean and fat	3 oz.	269	21	20
Leg, roasted Lean and fat	3 oz.	219	22	14
Rib, roasted Lean and fat	3 oz.	305	18	25
Pork, *cured, cooked* Bacon, regular	3 slices	109	6	9

Saturated fat (gm)	Cholesterol (mg)	Carbohydrates (gm)	Fiber (gm)	Sodium (mg)
9.9	71	0	0	54
4.2	61	00	50	54
5.2	77	0	0	54
5.3	73	0	0	855
0.5	12	Tr	0	984
8.4	102	0	0	61
8.4	85	0	0	65
5.9	79	0	0	56
10.9	82	0	0	62
3.3	16	Tr	0	303

Food	Amount	Calories	Protein (gm)	Total fat (gm)
Pork, *cured, cooked* (*cont'd*) Bacon, Canadian	2 slices	86	11	4
Ham, lean and fat	3 oz.	207	18	14
Pork, *fresh, cooked* Chop, loin Broiled, lean and fat	3 oz.	204	24	11
Pan-fried, lean and fat	3 oz.	235	25	14
Ham (leg), roasted Lean and fat	3 oz.	232	23	15
Rib roast, lean and fat	3 oz.	217	23	13
Ribs, lean and fat Backribs	3 oz.	315	21	25
Country-style	3 oz.	252	20	18
Spareribs	3 oz.	337	25	26
Shoulder cut Lean and fat	3 oz.	280	24	20

Saturated fat (gm)	Cholesterol (mg)	Carbohydrates (gm)	Fiber (gm)	Sodium (mg)
1.3	27	1	0	719
5.1	53	0	0	1,009
4.1	70	0	0	49
5.1	78	0	0	68
5.5	80	0	0	51
5	62	0	0	397
9.3	100	0	0	86
6.8	74	0	0	50
9.5	103	0	0	79
7.2	93	0	0	75

Food	Amount	Calories	Protein (gm)	Total fat (gm)
Sausages & luncheon meats Bologna, beef, & pork	2 oz.	180	7	16
Brown & serve, link	2 oz.	103	4	9
Canned luncheon meat Pork w/ham, canned	2 oz.	188	8	17
Chopped ham	2 slices	48	4	4
Cooked ham	2 oz.	104	10	6
Frankfurter (10/lb.) Beef & pork	1 frank	144	5	13
Beef	1 frank	142	5	13
Pork sausage Link	2 links	96	5	8
Patty	1 patty	100	5	8
Salami	2 slices	84	5	7
Vienna sausage	1 sausage	45	2	4

Saturated fat (gm)	Cholesterol (mg)	Carbohydrates (gm)	Fiber (gm)	Sodium (mg)
6.1	31	2	0	581
3.4	18	1	0	209
5.7	40	1	0	758
1.2	11	0	0	288
1.9	32	2	0	751
4.8	23	1	0	504
5.4	27	1	0	462
2.8	22	Tr	0	336
2.9	22	Tr	0	349
2.4	16	1	0	372
1.5	8	Tr	0	152

Food	Amount	Calories	Protein (gm)	Total fat (gm)
Veal, lean and fat Cutlet	3 oz.	179	31	5
Rib	3 oz.	194	20	12

MIXED DISHES & FAST FOODS

Food	Amount	Calories	Protein (gm)	Total fat (gm)
Mixed dishes Beef macaroni, frozen	1 package	211	14	2
Beef stew, can	1 cup	218	11	12
Chicken potpie, frozen	1 small pie	484	13	29
Chili con carne, w/beans, can	1 cup	255	20	8
Macaroni & cheese, can	1 cup	199	8	6
Meatless burger, frozen	1 patty	91	14	1
Pasta w/meatballs, can	1 cup	260	11	10
Spaghetti bolognese, frozen	1 package	255	614	3

Saturated fat (gm)	Cholesterol (mg)	Carbohydrates (gm)	Fiber (gm)	Sodium (mg)
2.2	114	0	0	57
4.6	94	0	0	78
0.7	14	33	4.6	444
5.2	37	16	3.5	947
9.7	41	43	1.7	857
2.1	24	24	8.2	1,032
3	8	29	3	1,058
0.1	0	8	4.3	383
4	20	31	6.8	1,053
1	17	43	5.1	473

Food	Amount	Calories	Protein (gm)	Total fat (gm)
Mixed dishes *(cont'd)*				
Spaghetti in tomato sauce, can	1 cup	192	6	2
Spinach soufflé	1 cup	219	11	18
Tortellini, frozen	¾ cup	249	11	6
Fast foods *Breakfast* **items**				
Biscuit w/egg, sausage		581	19	39
Croissant w/egg, cheese, bacon	1 croissant	413	16	28
Eng. muffin w/egg, cheese, Canadian bacon	1 muffin	289	17	13
French toast sticks	5 sticks	513	8	29
Hashed brown potatoes	½ cup	151	2	9
Pancakes w/butter, syrup	2 pancakes	520	8	14
Burrito w/beans and cheese	1 burrito	189	8	6

Saturated fat (gm)	Cholesterol (mg)	Carbohydrates (gm)	Fiber (gm)	Sodium (mg)
0.7	8	39	7.8	963
7.1	184	3	NA	763
2.9	34	38	1.5	279
15	302	41	0.9	1,141
15.4	215	24	NA	889
4.7	234	27	1.5	729
4.7	75	58	2.7	499
4.3	9	16	NA	290
5.9	58	91	NA	1,104
3.4	14	27	NA	583

Food	Amount	Calories	Protein (gm)	Total fat (gm)
Fast foods *(cont'd)*				
Burrito w/beans and meat	1 burrito	255	11	9
Cheeseburger Reg. size w/condiments Double patty	1 sandwich	417	21	21
Single patty	1 sandwich	295	16	14
Reg. size, plain Double patty	1 sandwich	457	28	28
Single patty	1 sandwich	319	15	15
Chicken filet, plain	1 sandwich	515	24	29
Chicken pieces, boneless, fried	6 pieces	319	18	21
Chile con carne	1 cup	256	25	8
Chimichanga, w/beef	1 chimi-changa	425	20	20
Coleslaw	¾ cup	147	1	11

Saturated fat (gm)	Cholesterol (mg)	Carbohydrates (gm)	Fiber (gm)	Sodium (mg)
4.2	24	33	NA	670
8.7	60	35	NA	1,051
6.3	37	27	NA	616
13	110	22	NA	636
6.5	50	32	NA	500
8.5	60	39	NA	957
4.7	61	15	0	513
3.4	124	22	NA	1,007
8.5	5	13	NA	267
1.6	5	13	NA	267

Food	Amount	Calories	Protein (gm)	Total fat (gm)
Fast foods *(cont'd)*				
Desserts				
Ice milk, vanilla	1 cone	164	4	6
Sundae, hot fudge	1 sundae	284	6	9
Enchilada w/cheese	1 enchilada	319	10	19
Fish sandwich, w/tartar sauce, cheese	1 sandwich	523	21	29
French fries	1 small	291	4	16
	1 medium	458	6	25
	1 large	578	7	31
Hamburger Reg. size, w/condiments Double patty	1 sandwich	576	32	32
Single patty	1 sandwich	272	12	10
Hot dog, plain	1 sandwich	242	10	15
Hot dog, w/chili	1 sandwich	296	14	13

Saturated fat (gm)	Cholesterol (mg)	Carbohydrates (gm)	Fiber (gm)	Sodium (mg)
3.5	28	24	0.1	92
5	21	48	0	182
10.6	44	29	NA	784
8.1	68	48	NA	939
3.3	0	34	3	168
5.2	0	53	4.7	265
6.5	0	67	5.9	335
12	103	39	NA	742
3.6	30	34	2.3	534
5.1	44	18	NA	670
4.9	51	31	NA	480

Food	Amount	Calories	Protein (gm)	Total fat (gm)
Fast foods *(cont'd)* Mashed potatoes	⅓ cup	66	2	1
Nachos, w/cheese sauce	6–8 nachos	346	9	19
Onion rings, fried	8–9 rings	276	4	16
Pizza (slice=⅛ of 12″ pizza) Cheese	1 slice	140	8	3
Meat & veg.	1 slice	184	13	5
Pepperoni	1 slice	181	10	7
Roast beef sandwich, plain	1 sandwich	346	22	14
Salad, tossed, w/chicken, no dressing	1½ cups	105	17	2
Salad, tossed, w/egg, cheese, no dressing	1½ cups	102	9	6
Shake Chocolate	16 oz.	423	11	12
Vanilla	16 oz.	370	12	10

Saturated fat (gm)	Cholesterol (mg)	Carbohydrates (gm)	Fiber (gm)	Sodium (mg)
0.4	2	13	NA	182
7.8	18	36	NA	816
7	14	31	NA	430
1.5	9	21	NA	337
1.5	21	21	NA	382
2.2	14	20	NA	267
3.6	51	33	NA	792
0.6	72	4	NA	209
3	98	5	NA	119
7.7	43	68	2.7	323
6.2	37	60	1.3	273

Food	Amount	Calories	Protein (gm)	Total fat (gm)
Fast foods *(cont'd)*				
Shrimp, fried	6–8 shrimp	454	19	25
Submarine sandwich (6″ long), w/oil & vinegar				
Cold cuts (w/lettuce, cheese, salami, ham, tomato, onion)		456	22	19
Roast beef (w/tomato, lettuce, mayo)		410	29	13
Tuna salad (w/mayo, lettuce)		584	30	28
Taco, beef	1 small	369	21	21
Taco salad (w/ground beef, cheese, taco shell)	1½ cups	279	13	15
Tostada (w/cheese, tomato, lettuce)				
w/beans & beef	1 tostada	333	16	17
w/guacamole	1 guacamole 1 tostada	181	6	23

Saturated fat (gm)	Cholesterol (mg)	Carbohydrates (gm)	Fiber (gm)	Sodium (mg)
5.4	200	40	NA	1,446
6.8	36	51	NA	1,651
7.1	73	44	NA	845
5.3	49	55	NA	1,293
11.4	56	27	NA	802
6.8	44	24	NA	762
11.5	74	30	NA	871
5	20	16	NA	401

Food	Amount	Calories	Protein (gm)	Total fat (gm)

POULTRY & POULTRY PRODUCTS

Food	Amount	Calories	Protein (gm)	Total fat (gm)
Chicken Fried in vegetable shortening, batter-dipped Breast	½ breast	364	35	18
Drumstick	1 drumstick	193	16	11
Thigh	1 thigh	238	19	14
Wing	1 wing	159	10	11
Roasted Breast	½ breast	142	27	3
Drumstick	1 drumstick	76	12	2
Thigh	1 thigh	109	13	6
Stewed, chopped	1 cup	332	43	17
Chicken liver	1 liver	31	5	1
Duck, roasted	½ duck	444	52	25

Saturated fat (gm)	Cholesterol (mg)	Carbohydrates (gm)	Fiber (gm)	Sodium (mg)
4.9	119	13	0.4	385
3	62	6	0.2	194
3.8	80	8	0.3	248
2.9	39	5	0.1	157
0.9	73	0	0	64
0.7	41	0	0	42
1.6	49	0	0	46
4.3	116	0	0	109
0.4	126	Tr	0	10
9.2	197	0	0	144

Food	Amount	Calories	Protein (gm)	Total fat (gm)
Turkey Dark meat	3 oz.	159	24	6
Light meat	3 oz.	133	25	3
Ground	4 oz. patty	193	22	11
Turkey giblets	1 cup	242	39	7
Poultry food products Chicken Canned, boneless	5 oz.	234	31	11
Frankfurter (10/lb.)	1 frank	116	6	9
Roll, light meat	2 oz.	90	11	4
Turkey Gravy & turkey	5 oz. package	95	8	4
Patties	2¼ oz. patty	181	9	12
Roast, boneless, seasoned, cooked	3 oz.	132	18	5

Saturated fat (gm)	Cholesterol (mg)	Carbohydrates (gm)	Fiber (gm)	Sodium (mg)
2.1	72	0	0	67
0.9	59	0	0	54
2.8	84	0	0	88
2.2	606	3	0	86
3.1	88	0	0	714
2.5	45	3	0	617
1.1	28	1	0	331
1.2	26	7	0	787
3	40	10	0.3	512
1.6	45	3	0	578

Food	Amount	Calories	Protein (gm)	Total fat (gm)

SOUPS, SAUCES, & GRAVIES

Soups
Canned, condensed
 Prepared w/milk

Food	Amount	Calories	Protein (gm)	Total fat (gm)
Clam chowder, New England	1 cup	164	9	7
Cr. of Chicken	1 cup	191	7	11
Cr. of Mushroom	1 cup	203	6	14
Tomato	1 cup	161	6	6
Prepared w/water				
Bean w/pork	1 cup	172	8	6
Beef broth, bouillon, consommé	1 cup	29	5	0
Beef noodle	1 cup	83	5	3
Chicken noodle	1 cup	75	4	2
Chicken & rice	1 cup	60	4	2
Clam chowder, Manhattan	1 cup	78	2	2

Saturated fat (gm)	Cholesterol (mg)	Carbohydrates (gm)	Fiber (gm)	Sodium (mg)
3	22	17	1.5	992
4.6	27	15	0.2	1,047
5.1	20	15	0.5	918
2.9	17	22	2.7	744
1.5	3	23	8.6	951
0	0	2	0	636
1.1	5	9	0.7	952
0.7	7	9	0.7	1,106
0.5	7	7	0.7	815
0.4	2	12	1.5	578

Food	Amount	Calories	Protein (gm)	Total fat (gm)
Soups *(cont'd)*				
Canned, condensed				
Prepared w/milk				
Cr. of chicken	1 cup	117	3	7
Cr. of mushroom	1 cup	129	2	9
Minestrone	1 cup	82	4	3
Pea, green	1 cup	165	9	3
Tomato	1 cup	85	2	2
Veg. beef	1 cup	78	6	2
Vegetarian veg.	1 cup	72	2	2
Canned, ready-to-serve, chunky				
Bean w/ham	1 cup	231	13	9
Chicken noodle	1 cup	175	13	6
Vegetable	1 cup	122	4	4
Canned, ready-to-serve, low-fat, reduced-sodium				
Chicken broth	1 cup	17	3	0

Saturated fat (gm)	Cholesterol (mg)	Carbohydrates (gm)	Fiber (gm)	Sodium (mg)
2.1	10	9	0.2	986
2.4	2	9	0.5	881
0.6	2	11	1	911
1.4	0	27	2.8	918
0.4	0	17	0.5	695
0.9	5	10	0.5	791
0.3	0	12	0.5	822
3.3	22	27	11.2	972
1.4	19	17	3.8	850
0.6	0	19	1.2	1,010
0	0	1	0	554

Food	Amount	Calories	Protein (gm)	Total fat (gm)
Soups *(cont'd)*				
Canned, ready-to-serve, low-fat, reduced-sodium				
Chicken noodle	1 cup	76	6	2
Chicken & rice	1 cup	116	7	3
Clam chowder, New England	1 cup	117	5	2
Lentil	1 cup	126	8	2
Minestrone	1 cup	123	5	3
Vegetable	1 cup	81	4	1
Dehydrated				
Unprepared				
Beef bouillon	1 packet	14	1	1
Onion	1 packet	115	5	2
Prepared w/water				
Chicken noodle	1 cup	58	2	1
Onion	1 cup	27	1	1
Home prepared, stock				
Beef	1 cup	31	5	Tr

Saturated fat (gm)	Cholesterol (mg)	Carbohydrates (gm)	Fiber (gm)	Sodium (mg)
0.4	19	9	1.2	460
0.9	14	14	0.7	482
0.5	5	20	1.2	529
0.3	0	20	5.6	443
0.4	0	20	1.2	470
0.3	5	13	1.4	466
0.3	1	1	0	1,019
0.5	2	21	4.1	3,493
0.3	10	9	0.3	578
0.1	0	5	1	849
0.1	0	3	0	475

Food	Amount	Calories	Protein (gm)	Total fat (gm)
Soups *(cont'd)* **Home prepared, stock**				
Chicken	1 cup	86	6	3
Fish	1 cup	40	5	2
Sauces *Home recipe* Cheese	1 cup	479	25	36
White, w/whole milk	1 cup	368	10	27
Ready-to-serve Barbecue	1 Tbsp.	12	Tr	Tr
Cheese	¼ cup	110	4	8
Hoisin	1 Tbsp.	35	1	1
Nacho cheese	¼ cup	119	5	10
Pepper or hot	1 tsp.	1	Tr	Tr
Salsa	1 Tbsp.	4	Tr	Tr
Soy	1 Tbsp.	9	1	Tr

Saturated fat (gm)	Cholesterol (mg)	Carbohydrates (gm)	Fiber (gm)	Sodium (mg)
0.8	7	8	0	343
0.5	2	0	0	363
19.5	92	13	0.2	1,198
7.1	18	23	0.5	885
Tr	0	2	0.2	130
3.8	18	4	0.3	522
0.1	Tr	7	0.4	258
4.2	20	3	0.5	492
Tr	0	Tr	0.1	124
Tr	0	1	0.3	69
Tr	0	1	0.1	871

Food	Amount	Calories	Protein (gm)	Total fat (gm)
Sauces *(cont'd)*				
Ready-to-serve				
Spaghetti, marinara, pasta	1 cup	143	4	5
Teriyaki	1 Tbsp.	15	1	0
Worcestershire	1 Tbsp.	11	0	0
Gravies, canned				
Beef	¼ cup	31	2	1
Chicken	¼ cup	47	1	3
Mushroom	¼ cup	30	1	2
Turkey	¼ cup	31	2	1

SUGARS & SWEETS

Food	Amount	Calories	Protein (gm)	Total fat (gm)
Candy				
Caramel				
Plain	1 piece	39	Tr	1
Choc.-flavored roll	1 piece	25	Tr	Tr
Carob	1 oz.	153	2	9
Chocolate, milk				
Plain	1 bar	226	3	14

Saturated fat (gm)	Cholesterol (mg)	Carbohydrates (gm)	Fiber (gm)	Sodium (mg)
0.7	0	21	4	1,030
0	0	3	Tr	690
0	0	3	0	167
0.7	2	3	0.2	325
0.8	1	3	0.2	346
0.2	0	3	0.2	342
0.4	1	3	0.2	346
0.7	1	8	0.1	25
Tr	0	6	Tr	6
8.2	1	16	1.1	30
8.1	10	26	1.5	36

Food	Amount	Calories	Protein (gm)	Total fat (gm)
Candy *(cont'd)*				
Chocolate, milk w/almonds	1 bar	216	4	14
w/peanuts (Mr. Goodbar)	1 bar	267	5	17
w/rice cereal (Nestle's Crunch)	1 bar	230	3	12
Chocolate chips Milk	1 cup	862	12	52
Semisweet	1 cup	805	7	50
White	1 cup	916	10	55
Choc.-coated raisins	10 pieces	208	5	13
Fudge, from recipe Chocolate Plain	1 piece	65	Tr	1
w/nuts	1 piece	81	1	3
Vanilla Plain	1 piece	59	Tr	1
w/nuts	1 piece	62	Tr	2

Saturated fat (gm)	Cholesterol (mg)	Carbohydrates (gm)	Fiber (gm)	Sodium (mg)
7	8	22	2.5	30
7.3	4	25	1.7	73
6.7	6	29	1.1	59
31	37	90	5.7	138
29.8	0	106	9.9	18
33	36	101	0	153
5.8	4	20	1.9	16
0.9	2	14	0.1	11
1.1	3	14	0.2	11
0.5	3	13	0	11
0.6	2	11	0.1	9

Food	Amount	Calories	Protein (gm)	Total fat (gm)
Candy *(cont'd)*				
Gummy candies				
Gumdrops	1 cup	703	0	0
Gummy bears	10 bears	85	0	0
Gummy worms	10 worms	286	0	0
Hard candy	1 piece	24	0	Tr
Jelly beans	10 large	104	0	Tr
Kit Kat	1 bar	216	3	11
M&M's				
Peanut	10 pieces	103	2	5
Plain	10 pieces	34	Tr	1
Milky Way	1 bar	258	3	10
Reese's Peanut Butter Cup	2 cups	243	5	14
Snicker's	1 bar	273	5	14
Starburst fruit chews	1 piece	20	Tr	Tr

Saturated fat (gm)	Cholesterol (mg)	Carbohydrates (gm)	Fiber (gm)	Sodium (mg)
0	0	180	0	80
0	0	22	0	10
0	0	73	0	33
0	0	6	0	2
Tr	0	26	0	7
6.8	3	27	0.8	32
2.1	2	12	0.7	10
0.9	1	5	0.2	4
4.8	9	44	1	146
5	2	25	1.4	143
5.1	7	34	1.4	152
0.1	0	4	0	3

182

Food	Amount	Calories	Protein (gm)	Total fat (gm)
Frosting, ready-to-eat				
Chocolate	1/12 package	151	Tr	7
Vanilla	1/12 package	159	Tr[c]	6
Frozen dessert (non-dairy)				
Fruit & juice bar	2½ oz.	63	1	Tr
Ice pop	2 oz.	42	0	0
Italian ices	½ cup	61	Tr	Tr
Gelatin dessert				
Regular	½ cup	80	2	0
Reduced-cal.	½ cup	8	1	0
Honey	1 Tbsp.	64	Tr	0
Jams & preserves	1 Tbsp.	56	Tr	Tr
Jellies	1 Tbsp.	54	Tr	Tr
Marshmallows	1 regular	23	Tr	Tr

Saturated fat (gm)	Cholesterol (mg)	Carbohydrates (gm)	Fiber (gm)	Sodium (mg)
2.1	0	24	0.2	70
1.9	0	26	Tr	34
0	0	16	0	3
0	0	11	0	7
0	0	16	0	5
0	0	19	0	57
0	0	1	0	56
0	0	17	Tr	1
Tr	0	14	0.2	6
Tr	0	13	0.2	5
Tr	0	6	Tr	3

Food	Amount	Calories	Protein (gm)	Total fat (gm)
Puddings				
Dry mix & 2% milk				
Chocolate				
Instant	½ cup	150	5	3
Vanilla				
Instant	½ cup	148	4	2
Ready-to-eat				
Regular				
Chocolate	4 oz.	150	3	5
Rice	4 oz.	184	2	8
Tapioca	4 oz.	134	2	4
Vanilla	4 oz.	147	3	4
Fat-free				
Chocolate	4 oz.	107	3	Tr
Tapioca	4 oz.	98	2	Tr
Vanilla	4 oz.	105	2	Tr
Sugar				
Brown				
Unpacked	1 cup	545	0	0
Unpacked	1 Tbsp.	34	0	0

Saturated fat (gm)	Cholesterol (mg)	Carbohydrates (gm)	Fiber (gm)	Sodium (mg)
1.6	9	28	0.6	417
1.4	9	28	0	406
0.8	3	26	1.1	146
1.3	1	25	0.1	96
0.7	1	22	0.1	180
0.6	8	25	0.1	153
0.3	2	23	0.9	192
0.1	1	23	0.1	251
0.1	1	24	0.1	241
0	0	141	0	57
0	0	9	0	4

Food	Amount	Calories	Protein (gm)	Total fat (gm)
Sugar *(cont'd)*				
White				
Granulated	1 cup	774	0	0
Granulated	1 tsp.	16	0	0
Powdered	1 cup	467	0	Tr
Powdered	1 Tbsp.	31	0	Tr
Syrup				
Choc.-flavored syrup/topping				
Thin type	1 Tbsp.	53	Tr	Tr
Fudge type	1 Tbsp.	67	1	2
Corn, light	1 Tbsp.	56	0	0
Maple	1 Tbsp.	52	0	Tr
Molasses	1 Tbsp.	47	0	0
Table blend, pancake				
Regular	1 Tbsp.	57	0	0
Reduced-cal.	1 Tbsp.	25	0	0

Saturated fat (gm)	Cholesterol (mg)	Carbohydrates (gm)	Fiber (gm)	Sodium (mg)
0	0	200	0	2
0	0	4	0	Tr
Tr	0	119	0	1
Tr	0	8	0	Tr
0.1	0	12	0.3	14
0.8	Tr	12	0.5	66
0	0	15	0	24
Tr	0	13	0	2
0	0	12	0	11
0	0	15	0	17
0	0	7	0	30

Food	Amount	Calories	Protein (gm)	Total fat (gm)
VEGETABLES & VEGETABLE PRODUCTS				
Alfalfa sprouts, raw	1 cup	10	1	Tr
Artichokes	1 cup	84	6	Tr
Asparagus, green Cooked from raw	4 spears	14	2	Tr
from frozen	4 spears	17	2	Tr
Canned	4 spears	14	2	Tr
Bamboo shoots, canned	1 cup	25	2	1
Beans Lima, frozen Fordhooks	1 cup	170	10	1
Baby limas	1 cup	189	12	1

Snap, cut
Cooked
  from raw
  Green
	1 cup	44	2	Tr

Yellow	1 cup	44	2	Tr

Saturated fat (gm)	Cholesterol (mg)	Carbohydrates (gm)	Fiber (gm)	Sodium (mg)
Tr	0	1	0.8	2
0.1	0	19	9.1	160
Tr	0	3	1	7
0.1	0	3	1	2
0.1	0	2	1.2	207
0.1	0	4	1.8	105
0.1	0	32	9.9	90
0.1	0	35	10.8	52
0.1	0	10	4	4
0.1	0	10	4.1	4

Food	Amount	Calories	Protein (gm)	Total fat (gm)
Beans *(cont'd)* Snap, cut from frozen Green	1 cup	38	2	Tr
Yellow	1 cup	38	2	Tr
Canned Green	1 cup	27	2	Tr
Yellow	1 cup	27	2	Tr
Beans, dry. *See* **Legumes, Nuts, & Seeds**				
Bean sprouts (mung) Raw	1 cup	31	3	Tr
Cooked	1 cup	26	3	Tr
Beets Slices, cooked	1 cup	75	3	Tr
Slices, canned	1 cup	53	2	Tr
Beet greens	1 cup	39	4	Tr
Black-eyed peas from raw	1 cup	160	5	1

Saturated fat (gm)	Cholesterol (mg)	Carbohydrates (gm)	Fiber (gm)	Sodium (mg)
0.1	0	9	4.1	12
0.1	0	9	4.1	12
Tr	0	6	2.6	354
Tr	0	6	1.8	339
Tr	0	6	1.9	6
Tr	0	5	1.5	12
Tr	0	17	3.4	131
Tr	0	12	2.9	330
Tr	0	8	4.2	347
0.2	0	34	8.3	7

Food	Amount	Calories	Protein (gm)	Total fat (gm)
Black-eyed peas *(cont'd)* from frozen	1 cup	224	14	1
Broccoli Raw Chopped	1 cup	25	3	Tr
Spear, 5″	1 spear	9	1	Tr
Flower cluster	1 floweret	3	Tr	Tr
Cooked from raw Chopped	1 cup	44	5	1
Spear 5″	1 spear	10	1	Tr
from frozen, chopped	1 cup	52	6	Tr
Brussels sprouts, cooked	1 cup	61	4	1
Cabbage, common varieties, shredded Raw	1 cup	18	1	Tr
Cooked	1 cup	33	2	1

Saturated fat (gm)	Cholesterol (mg)	Carbohydrates (gm)	Fiber (gm)	Sodium (mg)
0.3	0	40	10.9	9
Tr	0	5	2.6	24
Tr	0	2	0.9	8
Tr	0	1	0.3	3
0.1	0	8	4.5	41
Tr	0	2	1.1	10
Tr	0	10	5.5	44
0.2	0	14	4.1	33
Tr	0	4	1.6	13
0.1	0	7	3.5	12

Food	Amount	Calories	Protein (gm)	Total fat (gm)
Carrots Raw Whole (7½″)	1 carrot	31	1	Tr
Grated	1 cup	47	1	Tr
Cooked, sliced from raw	1 cup	70	2	Tr
from frozen	1 cup	53	2	Tr
Cauliflower Raw	1 cup	29	2	1
from frozen	1 cup	34	3	Tr
Celery Raw	1 stalk	6	Tr	Tr
Cooked	1 stalk	7	Tr	Tr
Chives, raw	1 Tbsp.	1	Tr	Tr
Cilantro, raw	1 tsp.	Tr	Tr	Tr
Coleslaw, home prep.	1 cup	83	2	3
Collards, chopped from raw	1 cup	49	4	1

Saturated fat (gm)	Cholesterol (mg)	Carbohydrates (gm)	Fiber (gm)	Sodium (mg)
Tr	0	7	2.2	25
Tr	0	11	3.3	39
0.1	0	16	5.1	103
Tr	0	12	5.1	86
0.1	0	5	3.3	19
0.1	0	7	4.9	32
Tr	0	1	0.7	35
Tr	0	2	0.6	35
Tr	0	Tr	0.1	Tr
Tr	0	Tr	Tr	1
0.5	10	15	1.8	28
0.1	0	9	5.3	17

Food	Amount	Calories	Protein (gm)	Total fat (gm)
Collards, chopped *(cont'd)* from frozen	1 cup	61	5	1
Corn, sweet yellow from raw	1 ear	83	3	1
from frozen	1 ear	59	2	Tr
Corn, canned Cream style	1 cup	184	4	1
Whole kernel	1 cup	-166	5	1
Cucumber, peeled	1 cup	14	1	Tr
Eggplant	1 cup	28	1	Tr
Endive, curly	1 cup	9	1	Tr
Garlic, raw	1 clove	4	Tr	Tr
Kale, chopped from raw	1 cup	36	2	1
from frozen	1 cup	39	4	1
Leeks	1 cup	32	1	Tr

Saturated fat (gm)	Cholesterol (mg)	Carbohydrates (gm)	Fiber (gm)	Sodium (mg)
0.1	0	12	4.8	85
0.2	0	19	2.2	13
0.1	0	14	1.8	3
0.2	0	46	3.1	730
0.2	0	41	4.2	571
Tr	0	3	0.8	2
Tr	0	7	2.5	3
Tr	0	2	1.6	11
Tr	0	1	0.1	1
0.1	0	7	2.6	30
0.1	0	7	2.6	20
Tr	0	8	1	10

Food	Amount	Calories	Protein (gm)	Total fat (gm)
Lettuce, raw Butterhead, as Boston types, head, 5″ diam.	1 head	21	2	Tr
Iceberg (Crisphead), head, 6″ diam.	1 head	65	5	1
Looseleaf, shredded	1 cup	10	1	Tr
Romaine or cos, shredded	1 cup	8	1	Tr
Mushrooms Raw, pieces/slices	1 cup	18	2	Tr
Cooked, pieces	1 cup	42	3	1
Canned, pieces	1 cup	37	3	Tr
Mushrooms, shiitake Cooked pieces	1 cup	80	2	Tr
Dried	1 mushroom	11	Tr	Tr
Mustard greens	1 cup	21	3	Tr
Okra, sliced, from raw	1 cup	51	3	Tr

Saturated fat (gm)	Cholesterol (mg)	Carbohydrates (gm)	Fiber (gm)	Sodium (mg)
Tr	0	4	1.6	8
0.1	0	11	7.5	49
Tr	0	2	1.1	5
Tr	0	1	1	4
Tr	0	3	0.8	3
0.1	0	8	3.4	3
0.1	0	8	3.7	663
0.1	0	21	6	6
Tr	0	3	0.4	Tr
Tr	0	3	2.8	22
0.1	0	12	8	Tr

Food	Amount	Calories	Protein (gm)	Total fat (gm)
Onions Raw Chopped	1 cup	61	2	Tr
Whole, medium	1 whole	42	1	Tr
Cooked	1 cup	41	1	Tr
Onion rings, 2"–3" diam.	10 rings	244	3	16
Parsley, raw	10 sprigs	4	Tr	Tr
Parsnips	1 cup	126	2	Tr
Peas, edible pod from raw	1 cup	64	5	Tr
Peas, green Canned	1 cup	117	8	1
Frozen	1 cup	125	8	Tr
Peppers Hot, chili, green or red	1 pepper	18	1	Tr
Jalapeño, canned	¼ cup	7	Tr	Tr

Saturated fat (gm)	Cholesterol (mg)	Carbohydrates (gm)	Fiber (gm)	Sodium (mg)
Tr	0	1	0.3	Tr
Tr	0	1	0.3	Tr
Tr	0	21	2.9	6
5.2	0	23	0.8	225
Tr	0	1	0.3	6
0.1	0	30	6.2	16
0.1	0	11	4.5	6
0.1	0	21	7	428
0.1	0	23	8.8	139
Tr	0	4	0.7	3
Tr	0	1	0.7	434

Food	Amount	Calories	Protein (gm)	Total fat (gm)
Peppers *(cont'd)* Sweet Green, raw	1 cup	40	1	Tr
Red, raw	1 cup	40	1	Tr
Cooked Green, Red	1 cup	38	1	Tr
Pimiento, canned	1 Tbsp.	3	Tr	Tr
Potatoes Baked, w/skin	1 potato	220	5	Tr
Boiled, peeled	1 potato	118	3	Tr
Scalloped from dry mix	1 cup	228	5	11
from home recipe	1 cup	211	7	9
Potato products, prepared Au gratin from dry mix	1 cup	228	6	10
from home recipe	1 cup	323	12	19
French-fried, frozen	10 fries	100	2	4

Saturated fat (gm)	Cholesterol (mg)	Carbohydrates (gm)	Fiber (gm)	Sodium (mg)
Tr	0	10	2.7	3
Tr	0	10	3	3
Tr	0	9	1.6	3
Tr	0	1	0.2	2
0.1	0	51	4.8	16
Tr	0	27	2.4	5
6.5	27	31	2.7	835
5.5	29	26	4.7	821
6.3	37	31	2.2	1,076
11.6	56	28	4.4	1,061
0.6	0	16	1.6	15

Food	Amount	Calories	Protein (gm)	Total fat (gm)
Potato products, prepared *(cont'd)*				
Hashed brown from frozen	1 patty	63	1	3
from home recipe	1 cup	326	4	22
Mashed from dehydrated flakes	1 cup	237	4	12
from home recipe	1 cup	162	4	1
Potato pancakes, home prepared	1 pancake	207	5	12
Potato puffs, frozen	10 puffs	175	3	8
Potato salad, home prepared	1 cup	358	7	21
Pumpkin, mashed	1 cup	49	2	Tr
Pumpkin, canned	1 cup	83	3	1
Radishes, raw	1 radish	1	Tr	Tr
Rutabagas, cooked	1 cup	66	2	Tr
Sauerkraut, canned	1 cup	45	2	Tr

Saturated fat (gm)	Cholesterol (mg)	Carbohydrates (gm)	Fiber (gm)	Sodium (mg)
1.3	0	8	0.6	10
8,5	0	33	3.1	501
7.2	29	32	4.8	697
0.7	4	37	4.2	636
2.3	73	22	1.5	386
4	0	24	2.5	589
3.6	170	28	3.3	1,323
0.1	0	12	2.7	2
0.4	0	20	7.1	12
Tr	0	Tr	0.1	1
Tr	0	15	3.1	34
0.1	0	10	5.9	1,560

Food	Amount	Calories	Protein (gm)	Total fat (gm)
Shallots, raw	1 Tbsp.	7	Tr	Tr
Soybeans, green, cooked	1 cup	254	22	12
Spinach Raw Chopped	1 cup	7	1	Tr
Leaf	1 leaf	2	Tr	Tr
Cooked from raw	1 cup	41	5	Tr
from frozen	1 cup	53	6	Tr
Squash Summer, all varieties Raw	1 cup	23	1	Tr
Cooked	1 cup	36	2	1
Winter, all varieties Baked	1 cup	80	2	1
Sweet potatoes Baked, w/skin	1 potato	150	3	Tr
Boiled, w/o skin	1 potato	164	3	Tr

Saturated fat (gm)	Cholesterol (mg)	Carbohydrates (gm)	Fiber (gm)	Sodium (mg)
Tr	0	2	0.2	1
1.3	0	20	7.6	25
Tr	0	1	0.8	24
Tr	0	Tr	0.3	8
0.1	0	7	4.3	126
0.1	0	10	5.7	163
Tr	0	5	2.1	2
0.1	0	8	2.5	2
0.3	0	18	5.7	2
Tr	0	35	4.4	15
0.1	0	38	2.8	20

Food	Amount	Calories	Protein (gm)	Total fat (gm)
Sweet potatoes *(cont'd)* Canned, mashed	1 cup	232	4	1
Tomatoes Raw Chopped/sliced	1 cup	38	2	1
Whole—cherry	1 cherry	4	Tr	Tr
Canned	1 cup	46	2	Tr
Sun-dried	1 piece	5	Tr	Tr
Tomato juice, canned, salt added	1 cup	41	2	Tr
Tomato products, canned Paste	1 cup	215	10	1
Puree	1 cup	100	4	Tr
Sauce	1 cup	74	3	Tr
Stewed	1 cup	71	2	Tr
Turnips, cooked	1 cup	33	1	Tr
Turnip greens from raw	1 cup	29	2	Tr

Saturated fat (gm)	Cholesterol (mg)	Carbohydrates (gm)	Fiber (gm)	Sodium (mg)
0.1	0	54	4.6	135
0.1	0	8	2	16
Tr	0	1	0.2	2
Tr	0	10	2.4	355
Tr	0	1	0.2	42
Tr	0	10	1	877
0.2	0	51	10.7	231
0.1	0	24	5	85
0.1	0	18	3.4	1,482
Tr	0	17	2.6	564
Tr	0	8	3.1	78
0.1	0	6	5	42

Food	Amount	Calories	Protein (gm)	Total fat (gm)
Turnip greens (cont'd) from frozen	1 cup	49	5	1
Vegetable juice cocktail, canned	1 cup	46	2	Tr
Vegetables, mixed Canned	1 cup	77	4	Tr
Frozen	1 cup	107	5	Tr
Water chestnuts, canned	1 cup	70	1	Tr

MISCELLANEOUS ITEMS

Food	Amount	Calories	Protein (gm)	Total fat (gm)
Baking powders Double-acting	1 tsp.	2	Tr	0
Low-sodium	1 tsp.	5	Tr	Tr
Baking soda	1 tsp.	0	0	0
Beef jerky	1 large piece	81	7	5
Catsup	1 Tbsp.	16	Tr	Tr
Celery seed	1 tsp.	8	Tr	1

Saturated fat (gm)	Cholesterol (mg)	Carbohydrates (gm)	Fiber (gm)	Sodium (mg)
0.2	0	8	5.6	25
Tr	0	11	1.9	653
0.1	0	15	4.9	243
0.1	0	24	8	64
Tr	0	17	3.5	11
0	0	1	Tr	488
Tr	0	2	0.1	5
0	0	0	0	1,259
2.1	10	2	0.4	438
Tr	0	4	0.2	178
Tr	0	1	0.2	3

Food	Amount	Calories	Protein (gm)	Total fat (gm)
Chili powder	1 tsp.	8	Tr	Tr
Chocolate, unsweetened, baking Solid	1 square	148	3	16
Liquid	1 oz.	134	3	14
Cinnamon	1 tsp.	6	Tr	Tr
Cocoa powder, unsweetened	1 Tbsp.	12	1	1
Cream of tartar	1 tsp.	8	0	0
Curry powder	1 tsp.	7	Tr	Tr
Garlic powder	1 tsp.	9	Tr	Tr
Horseradish, prepared	1 tsp.	2	Tr	Tr
Mustard, prepared, yellow	1 tsp.	3	Tr	Tr
Olives, canned Pickled, green	5 med.	20	Tr	2
Ripe, black	5 large	25	Tr	2

Saturated fat (gm)	Cholesterol (mg)	Carbohydrates (gm)	Fiber (gm)	Sodium (mg)
0.1	0	1	0.9	26
9.2	0	8	4.4	4
7.2	0	10	5.1	3
Tr	0	2	1.2	1
0.4	0	3	1.8	1
0	0	2	Tr	2
Tr	0	1	0.7	1
Tr	0	2	0.3	1
Tr	0	1	0.2	16
Tr	0	Tr	0.2	56
0.3	0	Tr	0.2	408
0.3	0	1	0.7	192

Food	Amount	Calories	Protein (gm)	Total fat (gm)
Onion powder	1 tsp.	7	Tr	Tr
Oregano, ground	1 tsp.	5	Tr	Tr
Paprika	1 tsp.	6	Tr	Tr
Parsley, dried	1 Tbsp.	4	Tr	Tr
Pepper, black	1 tsp.	5	Tr	Tr
Pickles, cucumber Dill	1 med. pickle	12	Tr	Tr
Fresh	3 slices	18	Tr	Tr
Pickle relish, sweet	1 Tbsp.	20	Tr	Tr
Pork skin/rinds	1 oz.	155	17	9
Potato chips Plain Salted	1 oz.	152	2	10
Unsalted	1 oz.	152	2	10
Barbecue flavor	1 oz.	139	2	9
Sour cream & onion flavor	1 oz.	151	2	10

Saturated fat (gm)	Cholesterol (mg)	Carbohydrates (gm)	Fiber (gm)	Sodium (mg)
Tr	0	2	0.1	1
Tr	0	1	0.6	Tr
Tr	0	1	0.4	1
Tr	0	1	0.4	6
Tr	0	1	0.6	1
Tr	0	3	0.8	833
Tr	0	4	0.4	162
Tr	0	5	0.2	122
3.2	27	0	0	521
3.1	0	15	1.3	168
3.1	0	15	1.4	2
2.3	0	15	1.2	213
2.5	2	15	1.5	177

216

Food	Amount	Calories	Protein (gm)	Total fat (gm)
Potato chips *(cont'd)* Reduced-fat	1 oz.	134	2	6
Fat-free	1 oz.	75	2	Tr
Salt	1 tsp.	0	0	0
Trail mix Regular	1 cup	707	21	47
Tropical	1 cup	570	9	24
Vanilla extract	1 tsp.	12	Tr	Tr
Vinegar Cider	1 Tbsp.	2	0	0
Distilled	1 Tbsp.	2	0	0
Yeast, baker's Dry, active	1 pkg.	21	3	Tr
Compressed	1 cake	18	1	Tr

Saturated fat (gm)	Cholesterol (mg)	Carbohydrates (gm)	Fiber (gm)	Sodium (mg)
1.2	0	19	1.7	139
Tr	0	17	1.1	185
0	0	0	0	2,325
8.9	6	66	8.8	177
11.9	0	92	10.6	14
Tr	0	1	0	Tr
0	0	1	0	Tr
0	0	1	0	Tr
Tr	0	3	1.5	4
Tr	0	3	1.4	5

Suggested Weights for Adults

| Height[1] | Weight in pounds[2] | |
	19 to 34 years	35 years and over
5'0"	[3]97–128	108–138
5'1"	101–132	111–143
5'2"	104–137	115–148
5'3"	107–141	119–152
5'4"	111–146	122–157
5'5"	114–150	126–162
5'6"	118–155	130–167
5'7"	121–160	134–172
5'8"	125–164	138–178
5'9"	129–169	142–183
5'10"	132–174	146–188
5'11"	136–179	151–194
6'0"	140–184	155–199
6'1"	144–189	159–205
6'2"	148–195	164–210
6'3"	152–200	168–216
6'4"	156–205	173–222
6'5"	160–211	177–228
6'6"	164–216	182–234

[1] Without shoes.
[2] Without clothes.
[3] The higher weights in the ranges generally apply to men, who tend to have more muscle and bone; the lower weights more often apply to women, who have less muscle and bone.
Credit: National Research Council

Daily Food Diary

Most of us eat more than we think, and more often. Sometimes we eat too much of one type of food, or not enough of another, creating a nutritional imbalance. Use this sample diary to record and evaluate

FIRST DAY

BREAKFAST

_____
_____
_____
_____
_____

LUNCH

_____
_____
_____
_____
_____

DINNER

_____
_____
_____
_____
_____

SNACKS

_____
_____
_____
_____
_____

Daily Food Diary

your food intake or to set up your own meal plans. Remember to include beverages and items used in food preparation, such as oils and butter.

SECOND DAY

BREAKFAST

_____
_____
_____
_____
_____

LUNCH

_____
_____
_____
_____
_____

DINNER

_____
_____
_____
_____
_____

SNACKS

_____
_____
_____
_____
_____

10-Week Progress Chart for Weight Loss

Weigh yourself once a week (for example, every Monday if you begin your diet on a Monday), on the same scale, at the same time of day, wearing approximately the same amount of clothing. The first entry in the chart would come at the end of one full week of following your program.

Starting Weight _____ Goal Weight _____

Starting Date _____ Goal Date _____

	WEIGHT	LOSS
Week 1	_____	_____
Week 2	_____	_____
Week 3	_____	_____
Week 4	_____	_____
Week 5	_____	_____
Week 6	_____	_____
Week 7	_____	_____
Week 8	_____	_____
Week 9	_____	_____
Week 10	_____	_____

Abbreviations Used in This Book

approx.	approximately
av.	average
c.	cup(s)
choc.	chocolate
diam.	diameter
ea.	each
fl.	fluid
gm.	gram(s)
IU	international unit
lb.	pound
lg.	large
mcg	microgram(s)
med.	medium
min.	minute
mg	milligram(s)
oz.	ounce(s)
pkg.	package
serv.	serving(s)
Tbsp.	tablespoon(s)
Tr	trace
tsp.	teaspoon(s)
w/	with
w/o	without

Guide to Equivalent Weights and Measures

By Volume (Liquid/Fluid)
1 cup = ½ pint   = 8 fluid ounces   = 237 milliliters
4 cups = 1 quart   = 32 fluid ounces   = 0.946 liter
4 quarts = 1 gallon = 128 fluid ounces = 3.785 liters

2 tablespoons = 1 fluid ounce = 30 milliliters
16 tablespoons = 1 cup = 237 milliliters
3 teaspoons = 1 tablespoon = 15 milliliters

⅓ cup = 5 tablespoons + 1 teaspoon
¾ cup = 12 tablespoons
⅞ cup = 14 tablespoons

By Weight (Avoirdupois)
1 ounce = 28.35 grams
3½ ounces = 100 grams
1 pound = 16 ounces   = 453.6 grams
1 kilogram = 1000 grams = 2.2 pounds

Commercial Canned Goods

Av. Net Weight	Approx. Cups
8 oz.	1
10½–12 oz.	1¼
14–16 oz.	1¾
16–17 oz.	2
1 lb. 4 oz. (20 oz.)	2½
1 lb. 13 oz. (29 oz.)	3½

Estimating Portion Sizes

	uncooked amount	cooked yield
beans, dry	1 cup	2 cups
rice	1 cup	3 cups
spaghetti, dry	2 oz.	1 cup
chicken		
breast	1	3 oz.
thigh or drumstick	1	2 oz.
pork or lamb chop	1	3 oz.
ground beef, lean	4 oz.	3 oz.

GLOSSARY

absorption, uptake of substances by a tissue, as of nutrients through the wall of the intestine.

additive, 1. a substance added directly to food during processing, as for preservation, coloring, or stabilization. **2.** something that becomes part of food or affects it as a result of packaging or processing, as debris or radiation.

Adequate Intake (UI), a recommended intake value that is assumed to be adequate based on estimates of nutrient intake by a group or groups of healthy people; used when a Recommended Daily Allowance cannot be determined.

agar or **agar-agar,** a gel prepared from the cell walls of various red algae, used in laboratories as a culture medium, in food processing as a thickener and stabilizer, and in industry as a filler, adhesive, etc.

albumin or **albumen,** any of a class of simple, sulfur-containing, water-soluble proteins that coagulate when heated, occurring in egg white, milk, blood, and other animal and vegetable tissues and secretions.

alimentary, 1. concerned with the function of nutrition; nutritive. **2.** pertaining to food.

alimentary canal, a tubular passage functioning in the digestion and absorption of food and the elimination of food residue, beginning at the mouth and terminating at the anus.

alkaloid, any of a large class of bitter-tasting, nitrogen-containing, alkaline ring compounds common in plants and including caffeine, morphine, nicotine, quinine, and strychnine.

allergen, any substance, usually a protein, that induces an allergic reaction in a particular individual.

alpha-tocopherol, VITAMIN E.

amino acid, any of a class of organic compounds that contains at least one amino group and one carboxyl group: the alpha-amino acids are the building blocks from which proteins are constructed. See also **essential amino acid.**

amylase, any of several digestive enzymes that break down starches.

analogue, a food made from vegetable matter, especially soybeans, that has been processed to taste and look like another food, as meat or dairy, and is used as a substitute for it.

anorectic also **anoretic, 1.** having no appetite. **2.** causing a loss of appetite. **3.** a substance, as a drug, causing loss of appetite.

anorexia nervosa, an eating disorder characterized by a fear of becoming fat, a distorted body image, and excessive dieting leading to emaciation.

anorexic, 1. a person suffering from anorexia or especially anorexia nervosa. **2.** anorectic.

antinutrient, a substance that interferes with the utilization of one or more nutrients by the body, as oxalate and phytate, which prevent calcium absorption.

antioxidant, an enzyme or other organic substance, as vitamin E or beta carotene, capable of counteracting the damaging effects of oxidation in animal tissues.

Apgar score, a quantitative evaluation of the health of a newborn, rating breathing, heart rate, muscle tone, etc., on a scale of 1 to 10.

ascorbic acid, a white, crystalline, water-soluble vitamin occurring naturally in citrus fruits, green vegetables, etc., and also produced synthetically, essential for normal metabolism: used in the prevention and treatment of scurvy, and in wound healing and tissue repair. Also called **vitamin C.**

aspartame, a white crystalline powder synthesized from amino acids that is many times sweeter than sucrose and is used as a low-calorie sugar substitute.

assimilation, the conversion of absorbed food into the substance of the body.

autophagia also **autophagy,** the maintenance of bodily nutrition by the metabolic breakdown of some bodily tissues.

avitaminosis, any disease caused by a lack of vitamins.

balanced diet, a diet consisting of the proper quantities and proportions of foods needed to maintain health or growth.

bariatrics, (used with a sing. v.) a branch of medicine that deals with the control and treatment of obesity and allied diseases.

basal metabolic rate, the rate at which energy is expended while fasting and at rest, calculated as calories per hour per square meter of body surface. *Abbr.:* BMR

basal metabolism, the minimal amount of energy necessary to maintain respiration, circulation, and other vital body functions while fasting and at total rest.

B complex, VITAMIN B COMPLEX.

beta carotene, the most abundant of various isomers of carotene that can be converted by the body to vitamin A.

BHA, butylated hydroxyanisole: an antioxidant used to retard rancidity in products containing fat or oil.

BHT, butylated hydroxytoluene: an antioxidant used to retard rancidity in products containing fat or oil.

bioavailability, the extent to which a nutrient or medication can be used by the body.

bioflavonoid, any of a group of water-soluble yellow compounds, present in citrus fruits, rose hips, and other plants, that in mammals maintain the resistance of capillary walls to permeation and change of pressure. Also called **vitamin P.**

biogenic, 1. resulting from the activity of living organisms, as fermentation. **2.** necessary for the life process, as food and water.

biological value, the nutritional effectiveness of the protein in a given food, expressed as the percentage used by the body of either the total protein consumed or the digestible protein available.

biotin, a crystalline, water-soluble vitamin of the vitamin B complex, present in all living cells. Also called **vitamin H.**

BMI, or **Body Mass Index,** a measure of body fat that is based on height and weight and applies to both adult men and women.

BMR, basal metabolic rate.

bulimarexia, BULIMIA (def. 1).

bulimia, 1. Also called **bulimia nervosa.** a habitual disturbance in eating behavior characterized by bouts of excessive eating followed by self-induced vomiting, purging with laxatives, strenuous exercise, or fasting. **2.** Also called **hyperphagia.** abnormally voracious appetite or unnaturally constant hunger.

caffeine, a white, crystalline, bitter alkaloid usually derived from coffee or tea, used medicinally as a stimulant.

caffeinism, chronic toxicity caused by excessive intake of caffeine, characterized by anxiety, irritability, palpitations, insomnia, and digestive disturbances.

calciferol, a fat-soluble, crystalline, unsaturated alcohol occurring in milk, fish-liver oils, etc., produced by ultraviolet irradiation of ergosterol and used as a dietary supplement, as in fortified milk. Also called **vitamin D$_2$.**

calcitriol, 1. a vitamin D compound derived from cholesterol, involved in the regulating and absorption of calcium. **2.** a preparation of this compound, used in the treatment of osteoporosis and bone fracture.

calcium, a silver-white divalent metal, combined in limestone, chalk, etc., occurring also in animals in bone, shell, etc. *Symbol:* Ca.

calcium propionate, a white, water-soluble powder used in bakery products to inhibit the growth of fungi.

calorie or **calory, 1. a.** Also called **gram calorie, small calorie.** an amount of heat exactly equal to 4,1840 joules. *Abbr.:* cal **b.** (usually cap.) kilocalorie. *Abbr.:* Cal **2. a.** a unit equal to the kilocalorie, used to express the heat output of an organism and the energy value of food. **b.** the quantity of food capable of producing such an amount of energy.

calorifacient, (of foods) producing heat.

carbo, 1. carbohydrate. **2.** a food having a high carbohydrate content.

carbohydrate, any of a class of organic compounds composed of carbon, hydrogen, and oxygen, including starches and sugars, produced in green plants by photosynthesis; important source of food.

carbo-loading, the practice of eating large amounts of carbohydrates for a few days before competing in a strenuous athletic event, as a marathon, to provide energy reserves in the form of glycogen.

carotene also **carotin,** any of three yellow or orange fat-soluble pigments found in many plants, especially carrots, and transformed into vitamin A in the liver; provitamin A.

carrageenan or **carrageenin,** a colloidal substance extracted from seaweed used chiefly as an emulsifying and stabilizing ingredient in foods and pharmaceuticals.

casein, a protein precipitated from milk, as by rennet, and forming the basis of cheese.

CFNP, Community Food and Nutrition Programs.

Chinese-restaurant syndrome, a reaction, as headache or sweating, to monosodium glutamate, sometimes added to food in Chinese restaurants.

chlorine, a halogen element; a heavy, greenish-yellow, incombustible, water-soluble, poisonous gas that is highly irritating to the respiratory organs; used for water purification and in the manufacture of chemicals. *Symbol:* Cl

chlorophyll or **chlorophyl,** the green pigment of plant leaves and algae, essential to their production of carbohydrates by photosynthesis.

cholecalciferol, VITAMIN D₃.

cholesterol, a sterol abundant in animal fats, brain and nerve tissue, meat, and eggs that functions in the body as a membrane constituent and as a precursor of steroid hormones and bile acids: high levels in the blood are associated with arteriosclerosis and gallstones.

choline, one of the B-complex vitamins, found in the lecithin of many plants and animals; maintains cell membranes, promotes healthy liver, nerve function, and memory.

chromium, a lustrous metallic element used in alloy steels for hardness. *Symbol:* Cr

cobalamin also **cobalamine,** VITAMIN B₁₂.

code dating, the practice of placing a code indicating the date and site of packaging on certain products, as canned goods.

cod-liver oil, an oil extracted from the liver of cod and related fishes, used as a source of vitamins A and D.

collagen, a strongly fibrous protein that is abundant in bone, tendons, cartilage, and connective tissue, yielding gelatin when denatured by boiling.

complex carbohydrate, a carbohydrate, as sucrose or starch, that consists of two or more monosaccharide units. Compare **simple carbohydrate.**

copper, a metallic element having a reddish brown color, used as an electrical conductor and in the manufacture of alloys. *Symbol:* Cu

cyclamate, any of several chemical compounds used as a non-caloric sweetening agent in foods and beverages; banned by the FDA in 1970 as a possible carcinogen.

cystine, a crystalline amino acid occurring in most proteins, especially the keratins.

defibered, (of food) having little or no natural fiber, typically as the result of commercial refining or processing.

degerm, 1. to rid of germs. **2.** to remove the germ or embryo from (a kernel of grain), usually through milling.

dehydrate, 1. to lose an abnormal amount of water from the body. **2.** to free (fruit, vegetables, etc.) from moisture for preservation; dry.

dehydration, 1. the act or process of dehydrating. **2.** an abnormal loss of water from the body, especially from illness or physical exertion.

desiccate, to preserve (food) by removing moisture; dehydrate.

dextroglucose, dextrose.

dextrose, the dextrorotatory form of glucose, occurring in fruits and in animal tissues and commercially obtainable from starch by acid hydrolysis.

DHA, docosahexaenoic acid: an omega-3 fatty acid present in fish oils.

diet, 1. food and drink considered in terms of qualities, composition, and effects on health. **2.** a particular selection of food, especially for improving a person's physical condition or to prevent or treat disease: *a low-fat diet.* **3.** such a selection or a limitation on the amount a person eats for reducing weight: *to go on a diet.* **4.** the foods habitually eaten by a particular person, animal, or group.

dietary fiber, fiber.

Dietary Reference Intakes (DRIs), a family of nutrient reference values; consists of the Recommended Dietary Allowance (RDA), the Estimated Average Requirement (EAR), the Adequate Intake (AI), and the Tolerable Upper Intake Level (UL); used to prevent nutrient deficiencies and to reduce the risk of chronic diseases such as osteoporosis, cancer, and cardiovascular disease.

dietetic, 1. pertaining to diet or to regulation of the use of food. **2.** prepared or suitable for special diets, especially those requiring a restricted sugar, salt, or caloric intake. **3. dietetics,** (used with a sing. v.) the science concerned with nutrition and food preparation.

dietitian or **dietician,** a person who is an expert in nutrition or dietetics.

digestion, 1. the process in the alimentary canal by which food is broken up physically, as by the action of the teeth, and chemically, as by the action of enzymes, and converted into a substance suitable for absorption and assimilation into the body. **2.** the function or power of digesting food.

digestive, 1. serving for or pertaining to digestion. **2.** promoting digestion. **3.** a substance promoting digestion.

digestive system, the system by which ingested food is acted upon by physical and chemical means to provide the body with absorbable nutrients and to excrete waste products: in mammals the system includes the alimentary canal extending from the mouth to the anus and the hormones and enzymes assisting in digestion.

D.R.V., (on food labels) Daily Reference Value: the amount of nutrients appropriate for one day.

dyspepsia also **dyspepsy,** deranged or impaired digestion; indigestion (opposed to eupepsia).

dyspeptic, 1. pertaining to, subject to, or suffering from dyspepsia. **2.** a person subject to or suffering from dyspepsia.

dystrophy also **dystrophia,** faulty or inadequate nutrition or development.

EDTA, ethylenediaminetetraacetic acid: a colorless compound capable of chelating a variety of divalent metal cations: used in food preservation, as an anticoagulant, and in the treatment of heavy metal poisonings.

empty calorie, a calorie whose food source has little or no nutritional value.

enrich, 1. to restore to (a food) a nutrient lost in processing. **2.** to add vitamins and minerals to (food) to enhance its nutritive value.

enzyme, any of various proteins, as pepsin and amylase, originating from living cells and capable of producing certain chemical changes in organic substances by catalytic action, as in digestion.

EPA, eicosapentaenoic acid: an omega-3 fatty acid present in fish oils.

esophagus, a muscular tube for the passage of food from the pharynx to the stomach; gullet.

essential amino acid, any amino acid that is required for life and growth but is not produced in the body, or is produced in insufficient amounts, and must be supplied by protein in the diet.

Estimated Average Requirement (EAR), a daily intake nutrient value that is estimated to meet the requirement of half of the healthy individuals in a life stage and gender group; used to assess dietary adequacy and as the basis for the Recommended Daily Allowance.

eupepsia, good digestion (opposed to dyspepsia).

eutrophy, healthy or adequate nutrition or development.

expiration date, the last date that a product, as food, should be used before it is considered spoiled or ineffective, usually specified on the label or package.

extender, a substance added to another substance, as to food, to increase its volume or bulk.

fat, 1. any of several oily substances that are the chief component of animal adipose tissue and many plant seeds. **2.** animal tissue containing much fat. **3.** obesity; corpulence.

fat-soluble, capable of dissolving in oil or fats.

fatty acid, any of a class of organic acids consisting of a long hydrocarbon chain ending in a carboxyl group that bonds to glycerol to form a fat.

FDA, Food and Drug Administration.

FD&C color, any of the synthetic pigments and dyes that are approved by the FDA for use in foods, drugs, and cosmetics.

fiber, the structural parts of plants, as cellulose, pectin, and lignin, that are wholly or partly indigestible, acting to increase intestinal bulk and peristalsis.

fish protein concentrate, an odorless and tasteless high-protein food additive made from ground fish and suitable for human consumption. *Abbr.:* FPC

fluoride, 1. a salt of hydrofluoric acid consisting of two elements, one of which is fluorine, as sodium fluoride. **2.** a compound containing fluorine.

fluorine, the most reactive nonmetallic element, a pale yellow, corrosive, toxic gas that occurs combined in minerals and is found naturally in bones and teeth. *Symbol:* F

folate, FOLIC ACID.

folic acid, a water-soluble vitamin that is converted to a coenzyme essential to purine and thymine biosynthesis: deficiency causes a form of anemia.

food additive, additive (def. 1).

food poisoning, 1. any illness, as salmonellosis or botulism, caused by eating food contaminated with bacterial toxins and typically marked by severe intestinal symptoms, as diarrhea, vomiting, and cramps. **2.** any illness caused by eating poisonous mushrooms, plants, fish, etc., or food containing chemical contaminants.

food science, the study of the nature of foods and the changes that occur in them naturally and as a result of handling and processing.

formula, 1. a recipe or prescription. **2.** a special nutritive mixture, especially of milk or milk substitute with other ingredients, in prescribed proportions for feeding a baby.

fortify, to add one or more ingredients to (a food) to increase its nutritional content.

freshness date, the last date, usually specified on the label or packaging, that a food, as bread, is considered fresh, although it may be sold, ordinarily at reduced prices, or eaten after that date.

fructose, a yellowish to white, crystalline, water-soluble, levorotatory ketose sugar sweeter than sucrose, occurring in invert sugar, honey, and a great many fruits: used in foodstuffs and in medicine chiefly in solution as an intravenous nutrient. Also called **levulose, fruit sugar.**

fruitarian, a person whose diet consists chiefly of fruit.

gliadin, a simple protein of cereal grains that imparts elastic properties to flour: used as a nutrient in high-protein diets.

glucose, a simple sugar that is a product of photosynthesis and is the principal source of energy for all living organisms: concentrated in fruits and honey or readily obtainable from starch, other carbohydrates, or glycogen.

gluten, a grayish, sticky component of wheat flour and other grain flours, composed mainly of the proteins gliadin and glutenin.

glutenin, a simple protein of cereal grains that imparts adhesive properties to flour.

glycerin also **glycerine, GLYCEROL.**

glycerol, a colorless liquid used as a sweetener and preservative, and in suppositories and skin emollients.

glycine, a sweet crystalline solid, the simplest amino acid, present in most proteins. *Abbr.:* Gly; *Symbol:* G

glycogen, a polysaccharide composed of glucose isomers that is the principal carbohydrate stored by the animal body and is readily converted to glucose when needed for energy use.

gorp, a mixture of nuts, raisins, dried fruits, seeds, or the like eaten as a high-energy snack, as by hikers and climbers.

granola, a breakfast food consisting of rolled oats, brown sugar, nuts, dried fruit, etc., usually served with milk.

GRAS, generally recognized as safe: a status label assigned by the FDA to a listing of substances (GRAS list) not known to be hazardous to health.

growth factor, any of various proteins that promote the growth, organization, and maintenance of cells and tissues.

growth hormone, any substance that stimulates or controls the growth of an organism, especially a species-specific hormone, as the human hormone somatotropin.

HDL, high-density lipoprotein.

health food, any natural food popularly believed to promote or sustain good health, as through its vital nutrients.

high-density lipoprotein, a circulating lipoprotein that picks up cholesterol in the arteries and deposits it in the liver for reprocessing or excretion. *Abbr.:* HDL

holism, an approach to healing or health care, often involving therapies outside the mainstream of medicine, in which isolated symptoms or conditions are considered secondary to one's total physical and psychological state.

holistic, 1. incorporating the concept of holism in theory or practice. **2.** identifying with principles of holism in a system of therapeutics, especially one considered outside the mainstream of scientific medicine, as naturopathy or chiropractic, and usually involving nutritional measures.

hormone, 1. any of various internally secreted compounds that are formed in endocrine glands and that affect the functions of specifically receptive organs or tissues when transported to them by the body fluids. **2.** a synthetic substance that acts like such a compound when introduced into the body.

human growth hormone, SOMATOTROPIN. *Abbr.:* hGH

HVP or **H.V.P.,** HYDROLYZED VEGETABLE PROTEIN.

hydrogenate, to combine or treat with hydrogen, esp. to add it to (an unsaturated organic compound).

hydrolyzed vegetable protein, a vegetable protein broken down into amino acids and used as a food additive to enhance flavor.

hyperphagia, BULIMIA (def. 2).

inositol, a compound occurring in animal tissue, plants, and many seeds, and functioning as a growth factor.

insulin, 1. a hormone, produced by the beta cells of the islets of Langerhans of the pancreas, that regulates the metabolism of glucose and other nutrients. **2.** any of several commercial preparations of this substance, each absorbed into the body at a particular rate: used for treating diabetes.

intestinal bypass, the surgical circumvention of a diseased portion of the intestine; also sometimes used to reduce nutrient absorption in morbidly obese patients.

intestine, 1. Usually, **intestines.** the lower part of the alimentary canal, extending from the pylorus to the anus. **2.** Also called **small intestine.** the narrow, longer part of the intestines, comprising the duodenum, jejunum, and ileum, that serves to digest and absorb nutrients. **3.** Also called **large intestine.** the broad, shorter part of the intestines, comprising the cecum, colon, and rectum, that absorbs water from and eliminates the residues of digestion.

invert sugar, a mixture of the dextrorotatory forms of glucose and fructose formed naturally in fruits and produced artificially by treating cane sugar with acids.

iodine, a nonmetallic halogen element occurring as a grayish-black crystalline solid that sublimes to a dense violet vapor when heated: used as an antiseptic and as a nutritional supplement. *Symbol:* I

iron, 1. a ductile, malleable, silver-white metallic element, used in its impure carbon-containing forms for making tools, implements, machinery, etc. *Symbol:* Fe **2.** a preparation of iron or containing iron, used chiefly in the treatment of anemia.

isoleucine, a crystalline amino acid occurring in proteins that is essential to the nutrition of humans and animals. *Abbr.:* Ile; *Symbol:* I

IV, an apparatus for intravenous delivery of electrolyte solutions, medicines, and nutrients.

junk food, food, as potato chips or candy, that is high in calories but of little nutritional value.

kwashiorkor, a disease, chiefly of children, caused by severe protein and vitamin deficiency and characterized by retarded growth, potbelly, and anemia.

lactarian, LACTOVEGETARIAN (def. 1).

lactase, an enzyme capable of breaking down lactose into glucose and galactose.

lactation, 1. the secretion of milk. **2.** the period of milk production.

lactobacillus, any of various anaerobic bacteria capable of breaking down carbohydrates to form lactic acid: cultured for use in fermenting milk into yogurt or other milk products.

lactogenic, stimulating lactation.

lacto-ovo-vegetarian, 1. Also called **lactovarian, ovolactarian, ovo-lacto-vegetarian.** a vegetarian whose diet includes dairy products and eggs. **2.** pertaining to or maintaining a vegetarian diet that includes dairy products and eggs.

lactose, a disaccharide present in milk that upon hydrolysis yields glucose and galactose.

lactovegetarian, 1. Also called **lactarian.** a vegetarian whose diet includes dairy products. **2.** pertaining to or maintaining a vegetarian diet that includes dairy products.

LDL, low-density lipoprotein.

lecithin, any of a group of phospholipids, containing choline and fatty acids, that are a component of cell membranes and are abundant in nerve tissue and egg yolk.

leucine, a white, crystalline, water-soluble amino acid obtained by the decomposition of proteins and made synthetically: essential in the nutrition of humans and animals. *Abbr.:* Leu; *Symbol:* L

levulose, fructose.

lipase, any of a class of enzymes that break down fats, produced by the liver, pancreas, and other digestive organs or by certain plants.

liquid protein, an amino acid hydrosol used in weight-reduction programs as a substitute for all or some meals: generally regarded as hazardous to health because of low nutritional content and recommended for controlled use only under medical supervision.

low-density lipoprotein, a plasma protein that is the major carrier of cholesterol in the blood, with high levels being associated with athero-sclerosis. *Abbr.:* LDL

lysine, a crystalline basic amino acid produced chiefly from many proteins by hydrolysis, essential in the nutrition of humans and animals. *Abbr.:* Lys; *Symbol:* K

macrobiotic, of or pertaining to macrobiotics.

macrobiotics, (used with a sing. v.) a program emphasizing harmony with nature, especially through a restricted, primarily vegetarian diet.

macromineral, any mineral required in the diet in relatively large amounts, especially calcium, iron, magnesium, phosphorus, potassium, and zinc.

macronutrient, any of the nutritional components required in relatively large amounts: protein, carbohydrate, fat, and the essential minerals.

magnesium, a ductile, silver-white metallic element that burns with a dazzling light. *Symbol:* Mg

malabsorption, faulty absorption of nutritive material from the intestine.

malassimilation, imperfect incorporation of nutrients into body tissue.

malnourished, poorly or improperly nourished; suffering from malnutrition.

malnutrition, lack of proper nutrition; inadequate or unbalanced nutrition.

maltose, a white, crystalline, water-soluble sugar formed by the action of diastase, especially from malt, on starch: used chiefly as a nutrient or sweetener, and in culture media. Also called **malt sugar.**

manganese, in nutrition, important for bone formation, metabolism of protein, fat, and carbohydrate; has antioxidant properties.

megavitamin, of, pertaining to, or using very large amounts of vitamins: *megavitamin therapy.*

menadione, a synthetic yellow crystalline powder, insoluble in water, used as a vitamin K supplement. Also called **vitamin K₃.**

metabolism, the sum of the physical and chemical processes in an organism by which its substance is produced, maintained, and destroyed, and by which energy is made available. Compare **anabolism, catabolism.**

metabolize, 1. to subject to or change by metabolism. **2.** to effect metabolism.

micronutrient, an essential nutrient, as a trace mineral, that is required in minute amounts.

mineral, any of the inorganic elements, as calcium, chromium, iron, magnesium, potassium, selenium, or sodium, that are essential to the functioning of the human body and are obtained from foods.

monosodium glutamate, a white, crystalline, water-soluble powder used to intensify the flavor of foods. Also called **MSG.** See also **Chinese-restaurant syndrome.**

monounsaturated, (of an organic compound) lacking a hydrogen bond at one point on the carbon chain.

monounsaturated fat, type of fat that is liquid at room temperature, found in vegetable oils, such as canola and olive oils; can help lower high blood cholesterol levels.

MSG, monosodium glutamate.

multivitamin, 1. containing or consisting of several vitamins. **2.** a compound of several vitamins.

natural, having undergone little or no processing and containing no chemical additives.

naturopathy, a method of treating disease that employs no surgery or synthetic drugs but uses fasting, special diets, massage, etc., to assist the natural healing processes.

neurotrophic, of or pertaining to the effect of nerves on the nutritive processes.

neurotrophy, the influence of the nerves on the nutrition and maintenance of body tissue.

niacin, nicotinic acid.

nicotinamide, a soluble crystal amide of nicotinic acid that is a component of the vitamin B complex and is present in most foods. Also called **niacinamide.**

nicotinic acid, a crystalline acid that is a component of the vitamin B complex, occurring in animal products, yeast, etc. Also called **niacin, vitamin B3.**

nitrite, SODIUM NITRITE.

nitrogen, a colorless, odorless, gaseous element that constitutes about four-fifths of the volume of the atmosphere and is present in combined form in animal and vegetable tissues, especially in proteins. *Symbol:* N

nourish, to sustain with food or nutriment; supply with what is necessary for life, health, and growth.

nourishment, something that nourishes; food, nutriment, or sustenance.

NutraSweet, *Trademark.* a brand of aspartame used in a low-calorie sweetener and in other processed foods, as soft drinks.

nutrient, 1. nourishing; providing nourishment or nutriment. **2.** containing or conveying nutriment, as solutions or vessels of the body. **3.** a nutrient substance.

nutrient-dense, (of food) relatively rich in nutrients for the number of calories contained.

nutriment, 1. any substance that, taken into a living organism, serves to sustain it, promoting growth, replacing loss, and providing energy. **2.** anything that nourishes; nourishment; food.

nutrition, 1. the study or science of the dietary requirements of humans and animals for proper health and development. **2.** the process by which organisms take in and utilize food material. **3.** food; nutriment.

nutritionist, a person who is trained or expert in the science of nutrition.

nutritious, providing nourishment, especially to a high degree; nourishing; healthful.

nutritive, 1. serving to nourish; nutritious. **2.** of, pertaining to, or concerned with nutrition. **3.** an item of nourishing food.

omega-3 fatty acid, a fatty acid found especially in fish oil and valuable in reducing cholesterol levels in the blood.

open dating, the practice of putting a freshness date on food packages.

organic, pertaining to, involving, or grown with fertilizers or pesticides of animal or vegetable origin, as distinguished from manufactured chemicals: *organic farming; organic fruits.*

overnutrition, the excessive intake of food, especially in unbalanced proportions.

ovolactarian, lacto-ovo-vegetarian.

ovo-lacto-vegetarian, lacto-ovo-vegetarian.

pancreas, a large compound gland, situated near the stomach, that secretes digestive enzymes into the intestine and glucagon and insulin into the bloodstream.

pancreatic juice, a colorless alkaline fluid secreted by the pancreas, containing enzymes that break down protein, fat, and starch.

pancreatin, a mixture of the pancreatic enzymes trypsin, amylase, and lipase, used to promote digestion.

pantothenic acid, a hydroxyl acid that is a component of the vitamin B complex, abundant in liver, yeast, and bran.

pepsin, 1. an enzyme, produced in the stomach, that splits proteins into proteoses and peptones. **2.** a commercial preparation containing pepsin, obtained from hog stomachs, used chiefly as a digestive and as a ferment in making cheese.

peptic, 1. pertaining to or associated with digestion; digestive. **2.** promoting digestion.

PGA, FOLIC ACID. [p(teroyl) + g(lutamic) a(cid)]

phenmetrazine, a compound used chiefly to control the appetite in the treatment of obesity.

phenylalanine, a crystalline, water-soluble, essential amino acid necessary to the nutrition of humans and most animals, occurring in egg white and skim milk. *Abbr.:* Phe; *Symbol:* F

phosphorus, a nonmetallic element existing in yellow, red, and black allotropic forms and an essential constituent of plant and animal tissue: used, in combined form, in matches and fertilizers. *Symbol:* P

phylloquinone, VITAMIN K₁.

phytonadione, VITAMIN K₁.

polyunsaturate, a type of fat found in vegetable oils that tends to lower cholesterol levels in the blood when substituted for saturated fats.

polyunsaturated, of or denoting a class of animal or vegetable fats, especially plant oils, whose molecules consist of carbon chains with many double bonds unsaturated by hydrogen atoms and that are associated with a low cholesterol content of the blood.

potassium, a silvery white metallic element: essential in metabolism and for maintenance of normal fluid balance. *Symbol:* K

predigest, to treat (food) by an artificial process analogous to digestion so that, when taken into the body, it is more easily digestible.

preservative, a chemical substance used to preserve foods or other organic materials from decomposition or fermentation.

protein, 1. any of numerous organic molecules constituting a large portion of the mass of every life form, composed of 20 or more amino acids linked in one or more long chains, the final shape and other properties of each protein being determined by the side chains of the amino acids and their chemical attachments. **2.** plant or animal tissue rich in such molecules, considered as a food source.

provitamin, a substance that an organism can transform into a vitamin, as carotene, which is converted to vitamin A in the liver.

provitamin A, CAROTENE.

PUFA, polyunsatured fatty acid.

pull date, the last date on which perishable food should be sold, usually established with some allowance for home storage under refrigeration. Also called **sell date.**

purine, a white, crystalline compound from which is derived a group of compounds including uric acid, xanthine, and caffeine.

pyridoxine also **pyridoxin,** a derivative of pyridine, required for the formation of hemoglobin and the prevention of pellagra; vitamin B₆.

Recommended Dietary Allowance (RDA), the average daily dietary intake level that is sufficient to meet the nutrient requirement of nearly all healthy individuals in a life stage and gender group.

Red No. 2, an artificial red dye used in foods, drugs, and cosmetics: banned by the FDA in 1976 as a possible carcinogen.

registered dietitian, a person who has fulfilled all the educational and examination requirements of the American Dietetic Association for recognition as a qualified nutrition specialist.

retinol, VITAMIN A.

riboflavin, a vitamin B complex factor essential for growth, occurring as a yellow crystalline compound abundant in milk, meat, eggs, and leafy vegetables and produced synthetically. Also called **vitamin B$_2$.**

saccharin, a white, crystalline, slightly water-soluble powder produced synthetically, which in dilute solution is 500 times as sweet as sugar: its soluble sodium salt is used as a non-caloric sugar substitute in the manufacture of syrups, foods, and beverages.

saturate, a saturated fat or fatty acid.

saturated fat, any animal or vegetable fat, abundant in fatty meats, dairy products, coconut oil, and palm oil, tending to raise cholesterol levels in the blood.

sea salt, table salt produced through the evaporation of seawater.

selenium, a nonmetallic element with an electrical resistance that varies under the influence of light. *Symbol:* Se

sell date, PULL DATE.

simple carbohydrate, a carbohydrate, as glucose, that consists of a single monosaccharide unit. Compare **complex carbohydrate.**

sitology, the branch of medicine dealing with nutrition and dietetics.

sodium, 1. a soft, silver-white, chemically active metallic element that occurs naturally only in combination: a necessary element in the body for regulating blood pressure and blood volume, as well as nerve and muscle function. *Symbol:* NA **2.** any salt of sodium, as sodium chloride or sodium bicarbonate.

sodium nitrate, a crystalline, water-soluble compound that occurs naturally as soda niter: used in fertilizers, explosives, and glass, and as a color fixative in processed meats.

sodium nitrite, a yellowish or white crystalline compound used as a color fixative and in food as a flavoring and preservative.

somatotropin, a polypeptide growth hormone of humans, secreted by the anterior pituitary gland. Also called **growth hormone.**

sorbitol, a sugar alcohol naturally occurring in many fruits or synthesized, used as a sugar substitute and in the manufacture of vitamin C.

stabilizer, any of various substances added to foods, chemical compounds, etc., to prevent deterioration, the breaking down of an emulsion, or the loss of desirable properties.

starch blocker or **starchblock,** a substance ingested in the belief that it inhibits the body's ability to metabolize starch and thereby promotes weight loss: declared illegal in the U.S. by the FDA.

sugar, 1. a sweet, crystalline substance obtained from the juice or sap of many plants, especially commercially from sugarcane and the sugar

beet; sucrose. **2.** any other plant or animal substance of the same class
  of carbohydrates, as fructose or glucose.
sulfite, any sulfite-containing compound, especially one that is used in
  foods or drug products as a preservative.
TDN t.d.n., totally digestible nutrients.
thiamine also **thiamin,** a crystalline, water-soluble vitamin-B compound abundant in liver, legumes, and cereal grains. Also called **vitamin B$_1$.**
tocopherol, any of several oils that constitute vitamin E.
Tolerable Upper Intake Level (UL), the highest level of daily nutrient intake that is likely to pose no risk of adverse health effects for almost all individuals in the general population.
total parenteral nutrition, intravenous administration of a solution
  of essential nutrients to patients unable to ingest food.
TPN, total parenteral nutrition.
trans fatty acids, fatty acids made through the process of hydrogenation, which solidifies liquid oils, increases the shelf life and flavor sta-
  bility of processed foods, and tend to raise blood cholesterol levels.
trophic, of or pertaining to nutrition; involving nutritive processes: *a
  trophic disease.*
TVP, *Trademark.* a brand of textured soy protein having various commercial uses as a meat substitute or extender.
undernourished, not nourished with sufficient or proper food to
  maintain health or normal growth.
undernutrition, nutritional deficiency resulting from lack of food or
  from the inability of the body to convert or absorb it.
uric acid, a compound present in urine in small amounts as the product
  of the metabolism of purines.
vegan, a vegetarian who omits all animal products from the diet.
vegetarian, 1. a person who does not eat meat, fish, fowl, or, in some
  cases, any food derived from animals. **2.** of or pertaining to vegetarianism or vegetarians.
vegetarianism, the practices or beliefs of a vegetarian.
vitamin, any of a group of organic substances essential in small quantities to normal metabolism, found in minute amounts in natural foodstuffs and also produced synthetically: deficiencies of vitamins
  produce specific disorders.
vitamin A, a yellow, fat-soluble alcohol obtained from carotene and occurring in green and yellow vegetables, egg yolk, etc.: essential to
  growth, the protection of epithelial tissue, and the prevention of night
  blindness. Also called **vitamin A$_1$, retinol.**
vitamin A$_2$, a yellow oil similar to vitamin A, obtained from fish liver.
vitamin B$_1$, THIAMINE.

vitamin B$_2$, RIBOFLAVIN.

vitamin B$_3$, NICOTINIC ACID.

vitamin B$_6$, PYRIDOXINE.

vitamin B$_{12}$, a complex water-soluble solid obtained from liver, milk, eggs, fish, oysters, and clams: a deficiency causes pernicious anemia and disorders of the nervous system. Also called **cobalamin.**

vitamin B complex, an important group of water-soluble vitamins containing vitamin B$_1$, vitamin B$_2$, etc.

vitamin C, ASCORBIC ACID.

vitamin D, any of the several fat-soluble vitamins occurring in milk and fish-liver oils, especially cod and halibut: essential for the formation of normal bones and teeth.

vitamin D$_1$, a form of vitamin D obtained by ultraviolet irradiation of ergosterol.

vitamin D$_2$, CALCIFEROL.

vitamin D$_3$, a form of vitamin D occurring in fish-liver oils that differs from vitamin D$_2$ by slight structural differences in the molecule. Also called **cholecalciferol.**

vitamin E, a pale-yellow viscous fluid, abundant in vegetable oils, whole-grain cereals, butter, and eggs, and important as an antioxidant in the deactivation of free radicals and in maintenance of the body's cell membranes: deficiency is rare. Also called **alpha-tocopherol.** Compare **tocopherol.**

vitamin G, RIBOFLAVIN.

vitamin H, BIOTIN.

vitamin K$_1$, a yellowish, oily, viscous liquid that occurs in leafy vegetables, rice, bran, and hog liver or is obtained especially from alfalfa or putrefied sardine meat or synthesized and that promotes blood clotting by increasing the prothrombin content of the blood. Also called **phylloquinone, phytonadione.**

vitamin K$_2$, a light yellow, crystalline solid having properties similar to those of vitamin K$_1$.

vitamin K$_3$, MENADIONE.

vitamin M, FOLIC ACID.

vitamin P, BIOFLAVONOID.

water-soluble, capable of dissolving in water.

xanthan, a gum produced by bacterial fermentation and used commercially as a binder or food stabilizer. Also called **xanthan gum.**

xanthine, a crystalline, nitrogenous compound related to uric acid, occurring in urine, blood, and certain animal and vegetable tissues.

yeast, 1. any of various small, single-celled fungi that reproduce by fission or budding and are capable of fermenting carbohydrates into alcohol and carbon dioxide. **2.** any of several yeasts used in brewing alcoholic beverages, as a leaven in baking breads, and in pharmacology as a source of vitamins and proteins.

Yellow No. 5, a yellow dye used in food, drugs, cosmetics, and other products: required by FDA regulations to be identified on food labels because of possible allergic reactions.

zinc, a ductile, bluish white metallic element: essential in minute quantities for physiological functioning. *Symbol:* Zn